Hips and Thighs

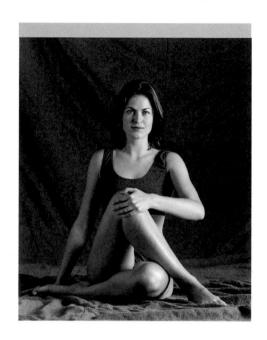

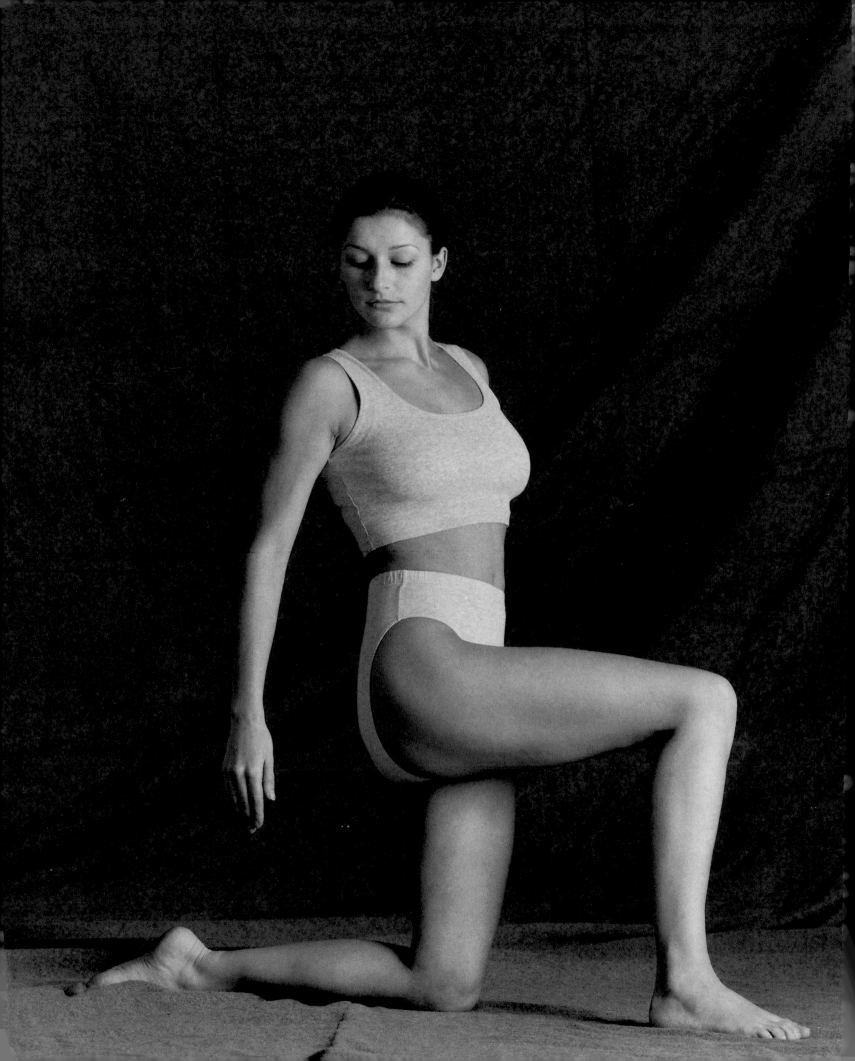

The Supple Workout

Hips and Thighs

Lorna Lee Malcolm

Photography by Antonia Deutsch

MACMILLAN • USA

MACMILLAN
A Simon and Schuster Macmillan Company
1633 Broadway
New York, NY 10019

A DBP Book
conceived, created and designed by
Duncan Baird Publishers
Sixth Floor
Castle House
75-76 Wells Street
London W1P 3RE

A catalogue record is available from the Library
of Congress.
ISBN 0-02-861346-5

Designers: Sue Bush, Gail Jones
Editor: Stephanie Driver
Commissioned Photography: Antonia Deutsch

10 9 8 7 6 5 4 3 2 1

Typeset in Frutiger
Colour reproduction by Bright Arts, Hong Kong
Printed in Singapore

Publishers' note
The exercises in this book are intended for
healthy people who want to be fitter. However,
exercise in inappropriate circumstances can be
harmful, and even fit, healthy people can injure
themselves. The publishers, DBP, the author, and
the photographer cannot accept any
responsibility for any injuries or damage
incurred as a result of using this book.

Contents

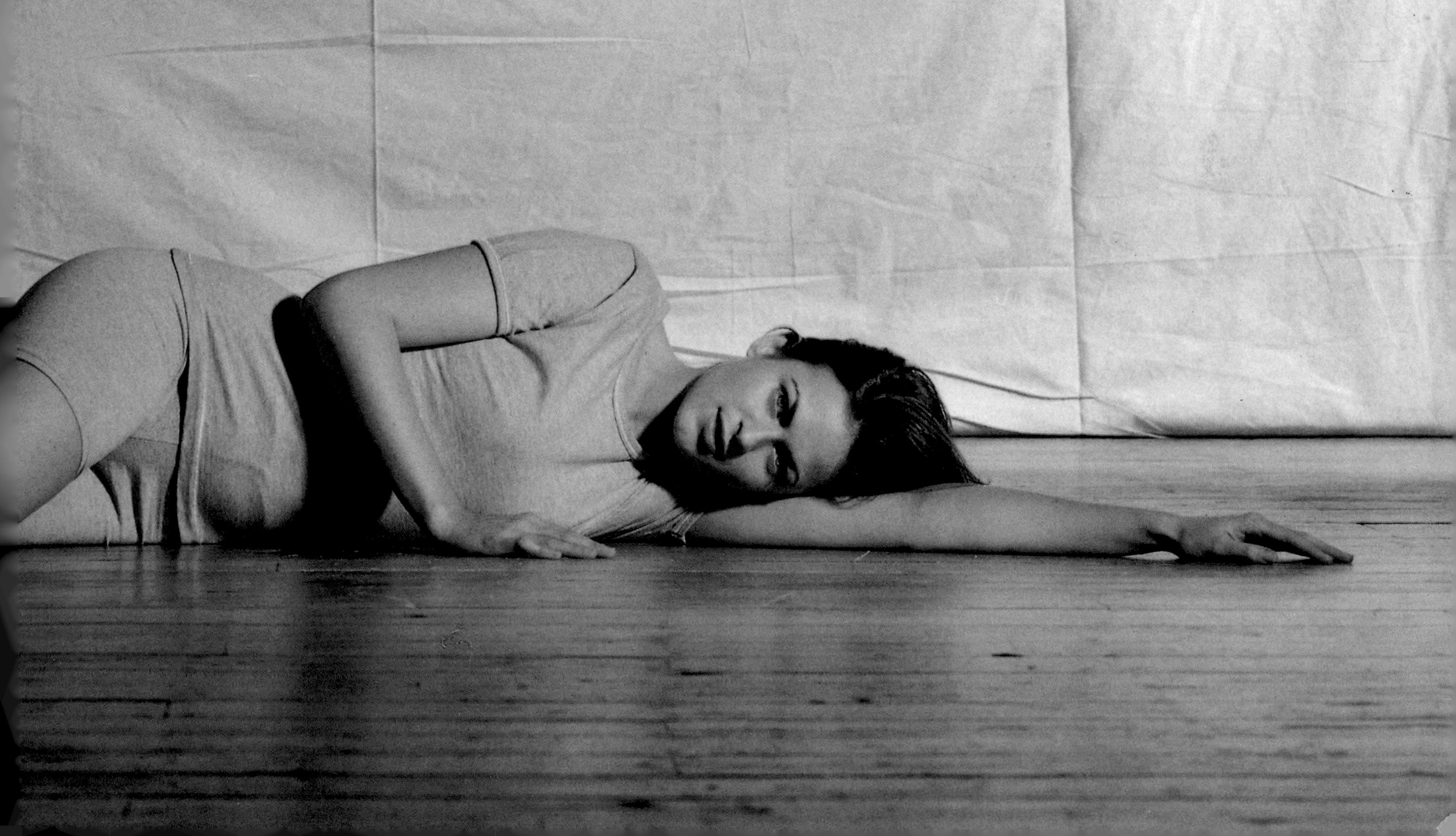

Introduction

For many of us, the hips and thighs are prime trouble-spots. Our modern, sedentary lifestyle means that we spend more time sitting than we do walking, and we take an elevator or an escalator more often than we climb stairs. When this is combined with a rich diet, our hips and thighs show the result – cellulite.

The solution is not difficult. An easy and enjoyable program of regular targeted exercise, combined with a healthy diet, will soon lead to a more toned and attractive body.

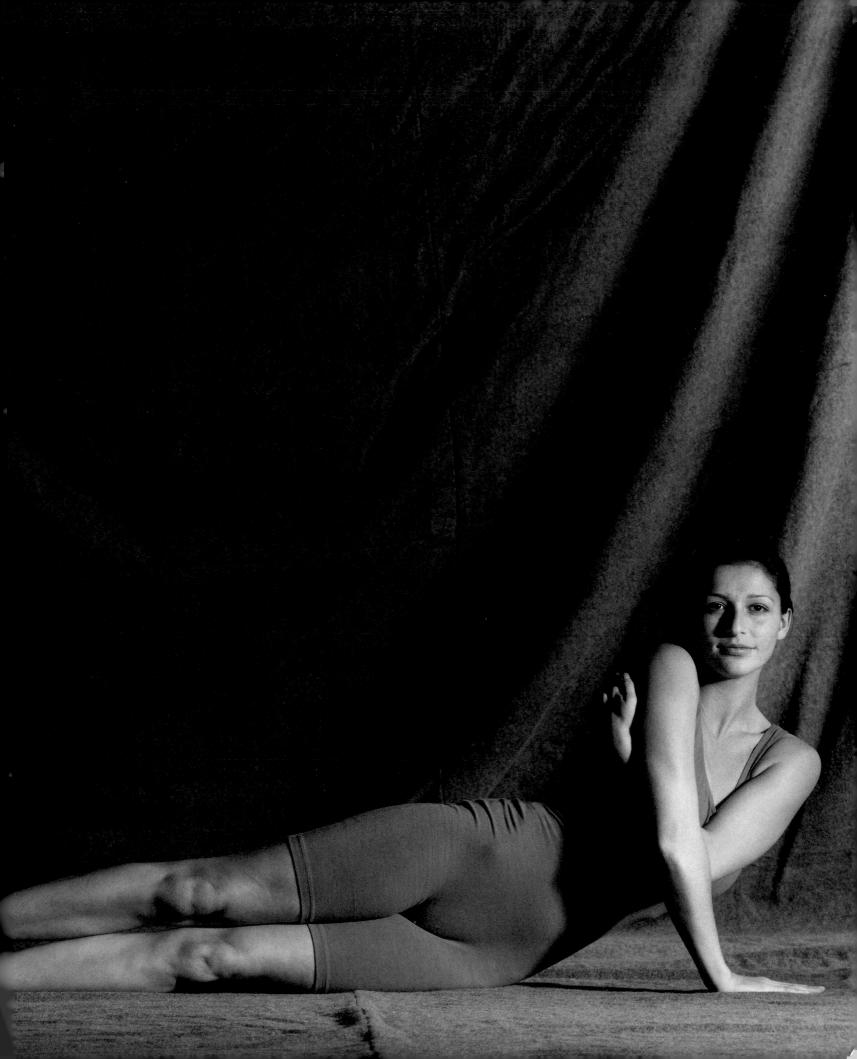

Getting started:
how to use this book

Exercise should be safe and effective, but it should also be fun. Don't let your workouts become a chore. Exercise with friends, play music, vary your format.

You know the saying, "go for the burn"? Well, ignore it. Exercise should make some demands on your body, because the body's response results in firmness and strength. But be aware of your body and how it feels. If you feel "the burn", stop immediately and gently stretch that area of your body to relieve the discomfort: you can also rub it gently.

Work gradually, especially if you have not done any exercise for some time. Always start with the simplest variation of an exercise. When more than one exercise has been given for the same muscle group, choose to focus on one or two at the most.

Change the exercises and the way you do them to keep variety in your exercise program, but remember that it takes your body some time to adapt to new demands. Follow a new routine for four to eight sessions before changing, and do a major reshuffle every four to six weeks to keep your body guessing and your muscles alert.

For support, choose a chair that is sturdy and a good height, so you can hold the back of it comfortably, without bending or tilting.

Enhance the exercises with weights. If you do not have hand weights, trying holding cans of beans or tomatoes. Water bottles are even better – you can fill them with sand, rice, or whatever is to hand. Start with the bottles half-full, gradually adding weight.

Each time you start, do a posture check –
• Center your weight over both feet.
• Stand tall without locking your knees.
• Have your hips in a neutral position, neither too far forward nor back.
• Pull in your abdominals and lengthen your spine. Imagine that your back and abdominal muscles are strong and solid, like a metal belt around your waist, so you can stabilize yourself from within, maintaining good posture and body alignment. Whenever you see the words "stabilize your torso" in this book, think of this metal belt.
• Lift your chest up and press your shoulders back and down to maximize lung capacity.
• Hold your neck long and aligned with your spine, and ease your head back so your chin does not protrude.

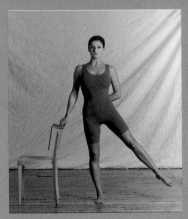

Core exercises, pages 22–39
These are the essential exercises for your hips and thighs. Organized by muscle group, they include both stretches and strength moves. To tone your hip and thigh area, you should try to do a selection of exercises from this section every other day.

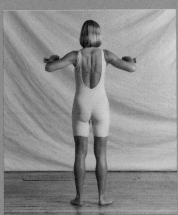

Warm-ups and cool-downs, pages 40–51
Before you begin to exercise, you should spend a few minutes warming up in order to get your muscles and joints moving freely, lessening the chance of injury. Similarly, you should devote time to the cool-down, gradually stretching the muscles you have worked and taking time to relax.

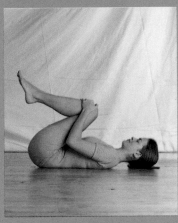

Total body workout, pages 52–67
These exercises covering the rest of the body complement the core exercises, so you can work toward overall health and fitness.

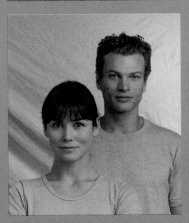

Routines, pages 68–77
In order to save time and keep yourself interested, you can combine exercises, developing a comprehensive workout covering your entire body. This section demonstrates key exercise combinations, giving you guidelines on how to devise your own.

Winning the war:
the fight against cellulite

Do women have to admit defeat in the war against cellulite? No, certainly not. With the correct approach, there is a lot you can do to improve the appearance of the areas where cellulite has developed. But the many expensive magic remedies on the market today may not offer the answers. The solution can be cheaper, easier, and much closer to home.

In order to understand how to improve the appearance of your hips and thighs, it helps to understand the physiology of your body.

In both men and women, fat makes up a percentage of our body weight, and it is stored throughout the body, not just in the places you most notice its appearance. The balance of hormones in a woman's body means that she has nearly twice the volume of fat, compared to an average man.

The distribution of fat on a woman's body is also different. It is to a large extent controlled by estrogen levels (estrogen is one of the most significant female sex hormones). Estrogen levels vary through our life cycle, which means that the way that our body distributes excess fat also varies. In your teens and 20s, excess weight is evenly distributed; in your 30s and 40s you tend to put it on your hips and thighs; and as you get older, you tend to put it on your waist.

The way in which the body stores fat is also determined hormonally. This is why women, unfortunately, suffer from cellulite and men in general do not.

Cellulite is not a different kind of fat – fat is fat. However, it has a different appearance in men than in women, particularly in certain notorious trouble spots, like the back of the thighs and the upper arms.

There is a marked difference in the structure of men's and women's skin, and especially in the connective tissue that runs between the layers of skin. This connective tissue builds chambers around which subcutaneous fat, the deeper layers of fat, are stored. In women the chambers created by connective tissue are more vertical than in men, so they are less adaptable to change. This means that when they become full, instead of bulging at the sides, the walls remain firm, and extra fat protrudes from the top. With age, the connective tissue becomes stronger and the

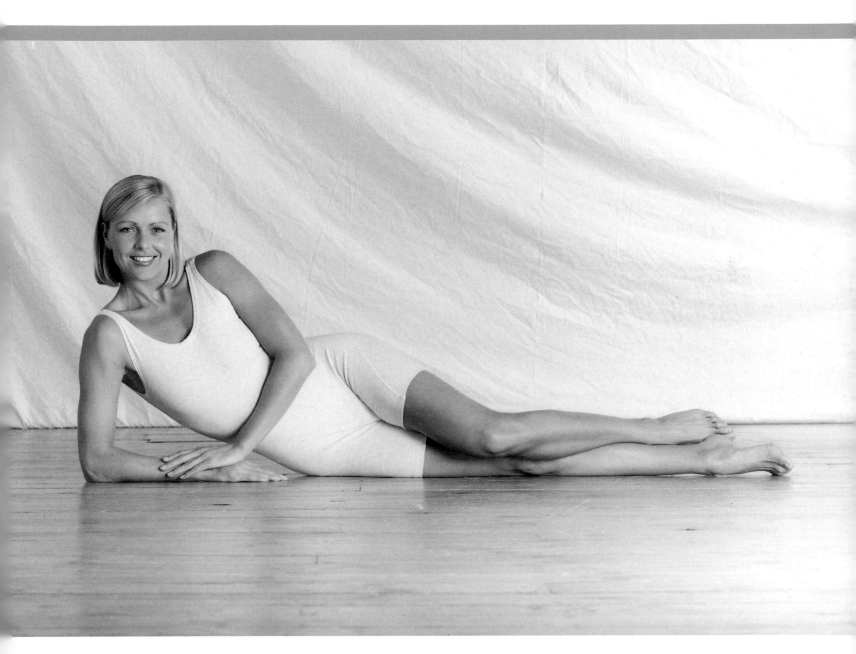

As you improve the muscle tone of your hips and thighs, you will find that they begin to appear firmer and more shapely.

skin becomes thinner, exaggerating the effect of cellulite. In men the connective tissue builds a structure akin to a honeycomb, which is a more flexible arrangement.

Many of the costly cellulite remedies marketed today, such as creams and massage mitts, will certainly help you to improve the condition of your skin. This is beneficial, since if your skin is firmer and smoother, the appearance of cellulite will lessen somewhat. However, these techniques have not been shown to have any effect on the underlying causes of the appearance of cellulite – they cannot change the structure of connective tissue, which is genetically determined, nor can they eliminate the fat stored in the body.

The only long-term solution to this age-old problem is exercise combined with a healthy diet. This will help tone and firm your hips and thighs. You will reduce the percentage of fat stored in your body by burning more energy than you take in with your diet.

Controlling the process

The combination of exercise and diet can also affect the way your body processes and stores fat in a more fundamental sense.

The way the body handles fat is determined by the levels of a number of hormones and enzymes. While much of this is out of our control, being part of the body's process of homeostasis, or internal self-regulation, we can take steps to control the ease with which the body stores, rather than uses, fat.

Diet is one line of defense. Cutting back on the amount of fat in your diet has two positive effects. One is, obviously, that if your body is supplied with less fat, it has less fat to store. It is also less likely to store the fat with which it is supplied, using it for essential metabolic processes instead.

Exercise is also your ally. You not only burn calories, helping you to balance your food intake with your body's needs, but you also reduce the activity of the enzymes that cause your body to store fat.

Be aware, however, that it is dangerous to cut too much fat from your diet. The human body needs a certain amount of fat and responds badly to being deprived: if you go on a "starvation" diet, totally cutting out fat (and therefore drastically limiting calories as well), your body will do all it can to conserve energy,

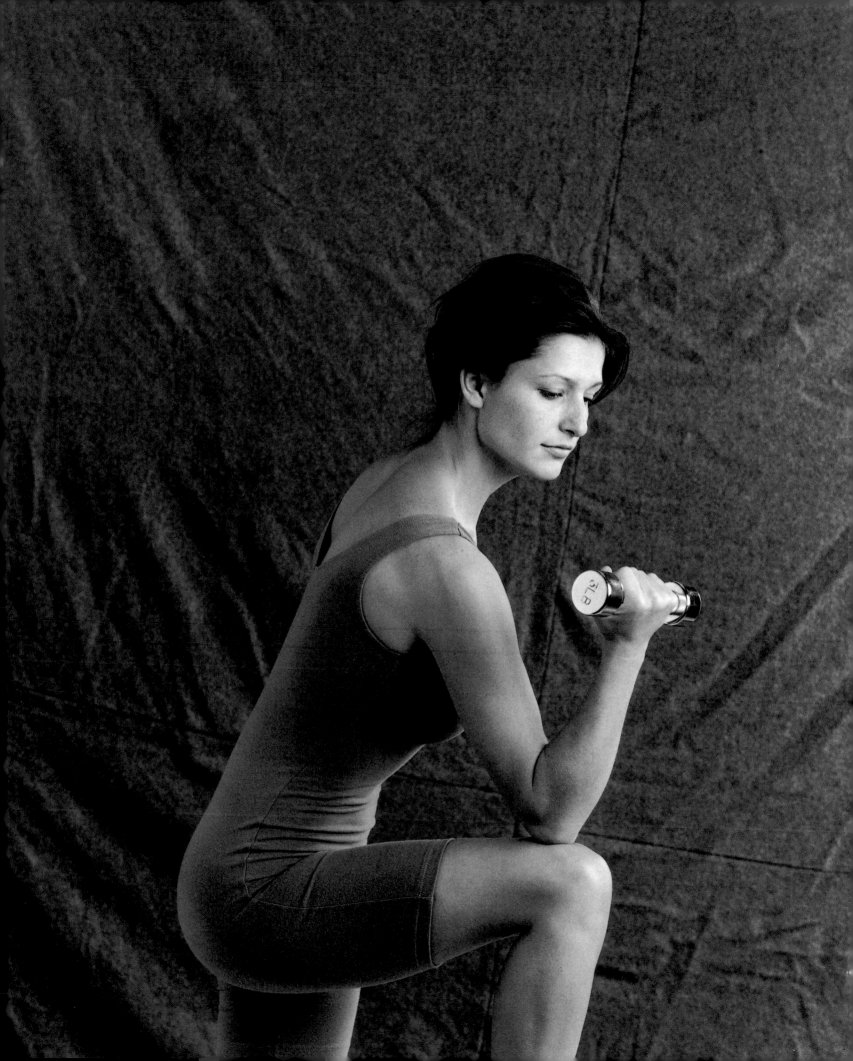

protecting its fat stores. This will make it harder to lose weight. In addition, excessive thinness carries its own dangers: it is linked to early death in both men and women, and to menstrual irregularity in women, which increases the risk of osteoporosis, or gradual weakening of the bones.

However, excess fat is also linked to a number of diseases, including heart disease and various forms of cancer in both men and women. If you are overweight, even a small weight loss, of only five or ten per cent of body weight can be enough to lessen the risk of these health problems.

If you ever feel dispirited, remember this little bit of good news. Some fat on the hips and thighs is actually good for you. Where you carry any excess weight also has ramifications for health. Studies have shown that a concentration of fat in the abdominal area is a greater health risk than a concentration of fat around the hips and thighs. This extra fat on the abdomen has been linked to certain types of cancer (including breast cancer and endometrial cancer), high blood pressure, heart disease and even diabetes. So beware of yo-yo dieting – the cycle of losing weight by

following strict diets, then putting the weight back on soon after. It can alter your natural distribution, causing you to gain weight on your abdomen.

Nor should you be seduced by the various detoxifying diet plans suggested specifically to tackle the problem of cellulite. Keep in mind that cellulite is a natural development in a woman's body – it does not result from an unnatural build-up of toxins. While a short, sensible detoxifying program may be revitalizing, it is not a long-term solution.

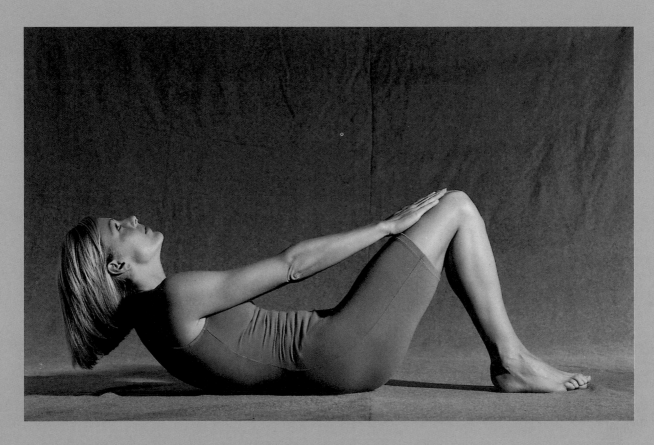

The right kind of targeted exercise, in combination with a healthy diet, will help you to improve the appearance of your hips and thighs, toning and firming these trouble spots.

Body facts

The muscles in the hips, thighs, and buttocks are some of the largest in the body, and also some of the hardest-working. They are integral in many of our regular activities, including walking, sitting, standing, and climbing stairs, so their condition is of prime importance to our overall fitness and health.

In order to tone these muscles effectively by stretching and strengthening them, it is important to understand where they are, how they are inter-related, and how they work.

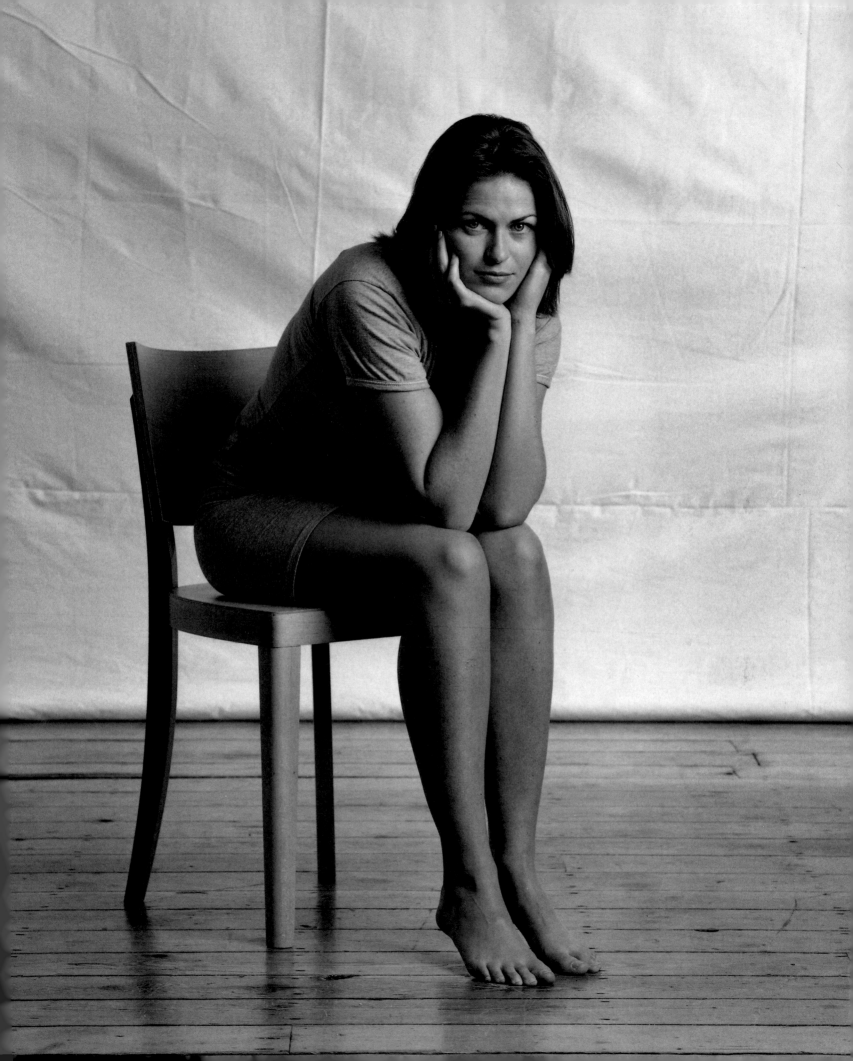

Body facts: hips, thighs, and buttocks

The muscles of the hips, thighs, and buttocks are some of the largest in the body and also some of the hardest-working. They are involved in many activities, including walking, climbing stairs, and sitting down and standing up. They are also integral in establishing the stability of the torso.

The intricate arrangement of the bones of the lower body means that we require very little actual muscle activity to stand upright – we are designed to balance.

The pelvic girdle – the correct name for the hipbones – connects the torso and legs, supports the internal organs, and balances the trunk. It consists actually of three bones, which fuse in early adulthood. A woman's pelvis is wider than a man's, to allow for the birth canal.

The muscles at the front of the thigh are known as the quadriceps and, as the name suggests, there are four parts to the group. At the top, three are directly attached to the femur, or thigh bone, and one is attached to the pelvis. At the lower end, the muscles form the patella tendon, which is attached to the kneecap. These muscles work to straighten your knees, and as part of that function, they also protect your knees by maintaining the position of your kneecaps.

Working in opposition to the quadriceps are the hamstrings, a group of three muscles in back of each thigh. This muscle group assists in straightening the body at the hip joint and in bending the knee. In most people, the hamstrings are smaller and weaker than the quadriceps. This imbalance means that they are more prone to injury. In addition, tightness in the hamstrings reduces the mobility of the hip joint, increasing strain on the lower back.

While all the muscles in our legs suffer from a sedentary lifestyle, the hamstring muscles suffer most from the inactivity. They shorten, making them tight, less efficient, and more prone to injury. It is essential to stretch this muscle group carefully during your warm-up not only when you run or play any sports, but also when you exercise at home.

It also is a good idea occasionally to focus specifically on your hamstring muscles (see pages 36–7) during workouts when you are working on your hips and thighs.

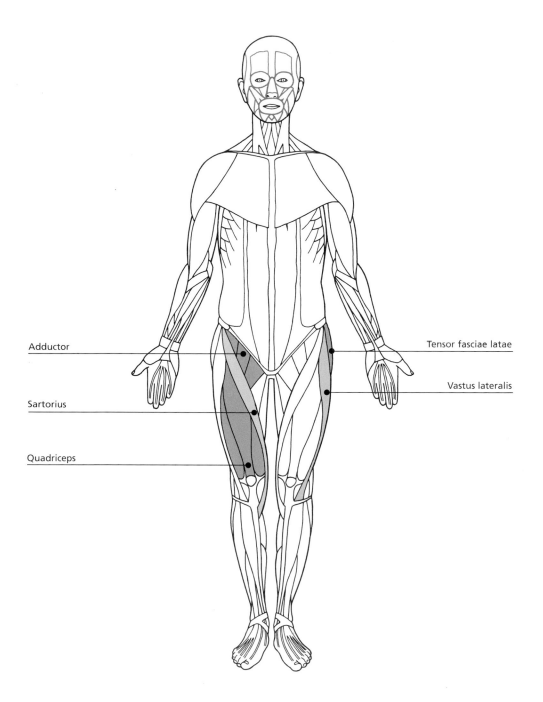

Adductor

Sartorius

Quadriceps

Tensor fasciae latae

Vastus lateralis

Front of the body

The quadriceps are the major muscles at the front of the thigh. It is a group of four muscles: three are attached directly to the thighbone and one is attached to the pelvic girdle (the hipbones). All four attach to the patella tendon, which connects to the kneecaps. The other muscles at the front of the thigh work to move your legs laterally, or sideways: the adductors move the leg toward the midline of the body and the abductors, the muscles on the outside of the thigh, move the leg *away.*

Just as the muscles of the front and back of the thigh work in opposition, so do the muscles of the inner and outer thigh. The outer thigh muscles are known as the abductors. These lift or move your legs laterally away from the midline of your body. The inner thigh muscles are known as the adductors, and they work to bring your legs together and to move them across the midline of the body when necessary. They attach the front of the pelvis to the femur, stabilizing the torso when you walk.

The hip flexors are the muscles that work specifically when you bend at the hip – for example, when you sit down or when you climb a step. Tight hip flexors can cause your back to arch excessively as the upper body is pulled forward constantly.

The main muscle of the buttocks, the gluteus maximus, is the largest in the body, and it forms the shape of the buttocks. Working in opposition to the hip flexors, this muscle is active when you straighten up at the hip joint – for example, when you climb stairs or when you stand up from sitting.

The hip joint is a ball-and-socket joint, like the shoulder. This means that it is designed for rotational motion, although its range of motion is more restricted than that of the shoulder. It is more flexible in bending forward than it is in bending backward, helping to ensure our stability when we are standing. This rotational motion is necessary for walking: when your right foot touches the ground in walking, the right hip joint rotates externally at the same time as the left hip joint rotates internally. The hip rotators, along with the gluteus muscles, are designed to control this rotational movement.

One of the reasons it is important to keep the muscles of the hips and thighs in good condition is that the hip joint bears a lot of force when you are walking or running. The muscles have to support the joint adequately, allowing it to bear the force more easily by taking advantage of its full range of motion.

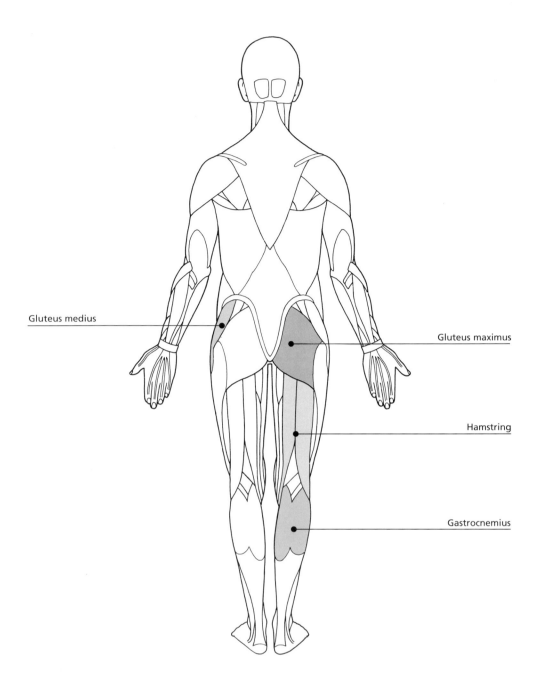

Gluteus medius

Gluteus maximus

Hamstring

Gastrocnemius

Back of the body

The gluteus maximus is the largest muscle in the body and forms the shape of the buttocks. Appearance is not the only reason to keep that muscle in shape: it is also involved in many activities, including climbing stairs and standing up from a sitting position.

The hamstring muscles are the major muscles of the rear thigh. In many people, they are shortened owing to inactivity and wearing high-heeled or restrictive shoes, and can therefore be uncomfortable. The same may be true of the gastrocnemius, the calf muscle.

Core exercises

These core exercises have been designed to work all the major muscle groups of the hips and thighs in a balanced manner, focusing on both stretch and strength. This way, your muscles can become firmer and tighter without growing bulky – stretching will help your muscles retain their length and take on a more desirable shape.

Balance your exercises between opposing body parts. For example, if you choose a strength exercise for the outer thigh, you should choose one for the inner thigh. You should also complement each strength exercise with a stretch to relax the muscles.

Don't expect immediate results – it takes the body six to eight weeks to adapt. Try to do this type of workout at least twice a week, aiming for a total time of 60 to 75 minutes. However, if 20 to 30 minutes is all you can spare, go for it anyway.

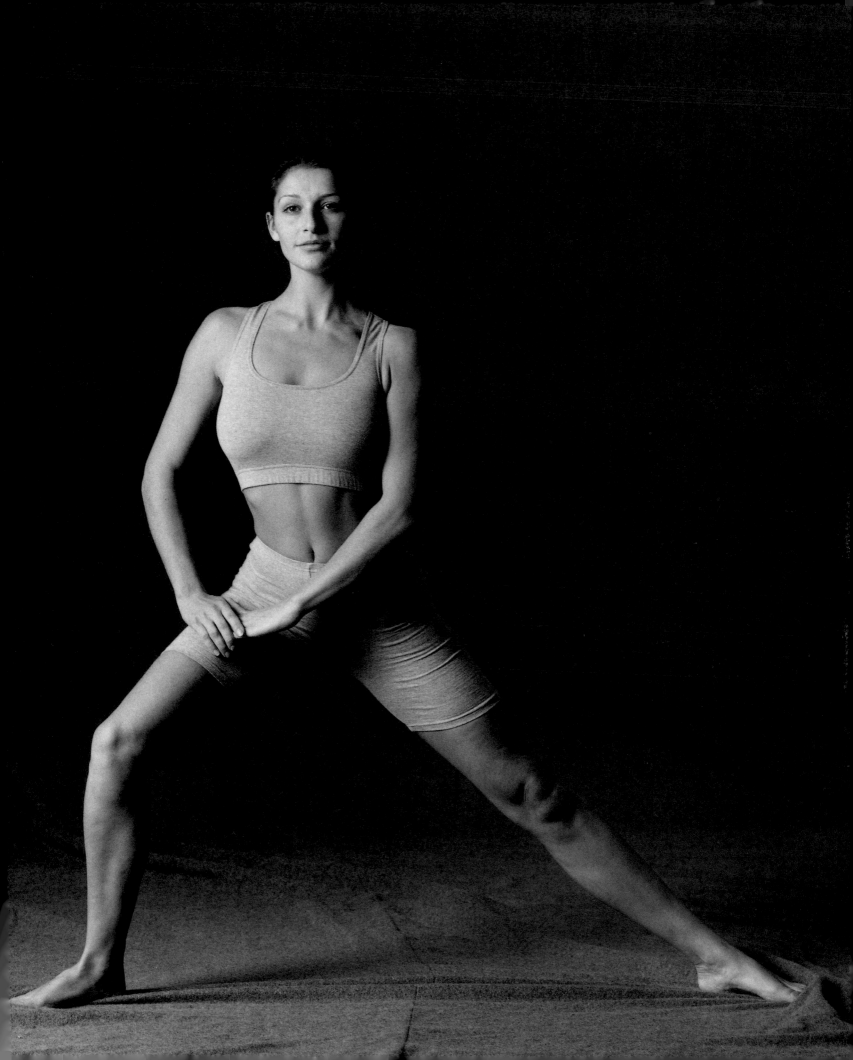

Outer thigh

The outer thigh muscles, or abductors, move your leg sideways away from the midline of your body, so to strengthen those muscles, you must move the leg in that direction, lifting the working leg to a 45° angle. Start at a slow pace, perhaps four beats to lift and four beats to lower, but you can vary this rhythm – it is more challenging to work slowly.

You can do this kind of exercise from a variety of positions: standing, kneeling, or lying. The kneeling position is the most advanced because it requires a lot of abdominal and back strength. If you try this and feel any strain, especially in your lower back, try one of the other options.

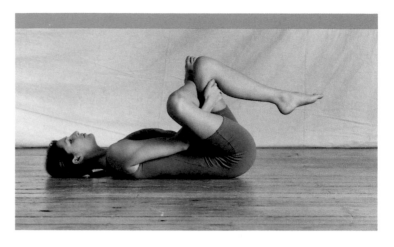

Heel-on-thigh stretch
Lie on your back with your left knee bent and your left foot on the floor. Rest the heel of your right foot on the thigh of your left leg so your right knee is pointing out to the right side. Keeping your left knee bent and your head and shoulders relaxed and on the floor, place both hands around your left thigh and pull it up and in toward your chest. You should feel a stretch along the right outer thigh. Hold this for at least 20 seconds.

Cross-legged stretch
Standing tall, cross your left foot closely behind your right foot, keeping both feet flat on the floor and the outside edges of your feet touching (1). Bend your right knee and, keeping your left leg straight, push your left hip out to the left side until you feel a stretch in your left buttock and along your left thigh (2). Although pushing out your hip will cause your torso to lean slightly in the opposite direction, try to keep your torso as long and strong as you can.

❶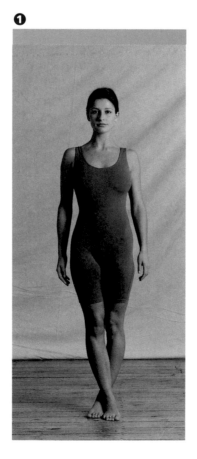

❷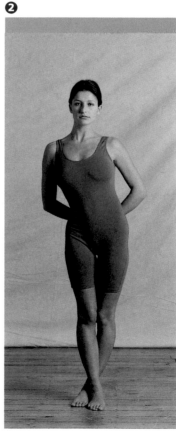

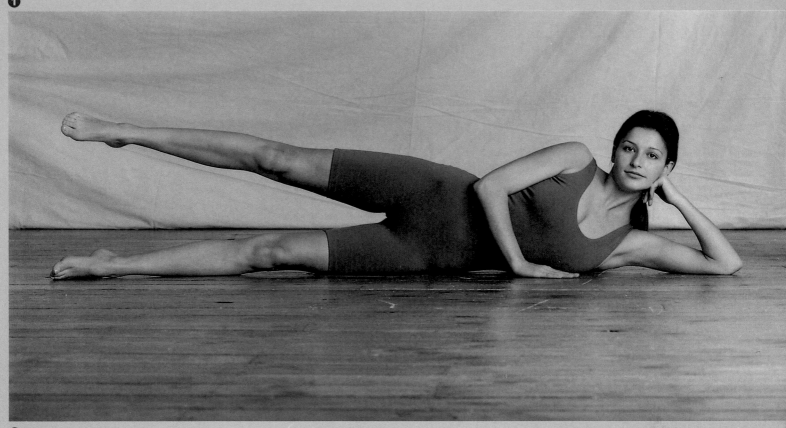

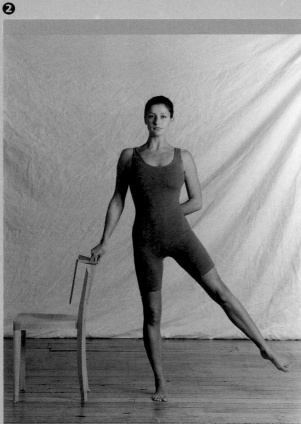

Side leg lift

Lie on your left side, keeping your body as long and extended as possible and making sure that your right hip is directly above your left hip. Place your right hand on the floor close to your chest to stabilize yourself. With a controlled movement, lift and lower your right leg as many times as you can, working toward at least 20 repetitions (1). To enhance the effectiveness of this exercise, lower your right leg to just above your left leg and immediately start the next lift, keeping a little tension in the muscles of your right leg through the movement.

You can also do this exercise while standing, using a chair or the wall as support (2). Remember to make sure that your hips are facing forward and your body is upright.

As an advanced variation, you can use ankle weights for added resistance.

Inner thigh

Your inner thigh muscles, known as adductors, work to bring your legs together and, if necessary, to move them past the midline of your body. These muscles may be stronger than the abductors of your outer thigh, because they are used more often. In order to tone the adductors, you have to repeat their usual movement but working against the downward force of gravity. This is the same principle applied to exercises to tone and strengthen the outer thighs.

To keep yourself motivated, you can vary the positions, doing these exercises standing, lying, or kneeling – standing is the easiest option, and kneeling is the most difficult. Aim to do at least 20 repetitions without resting.

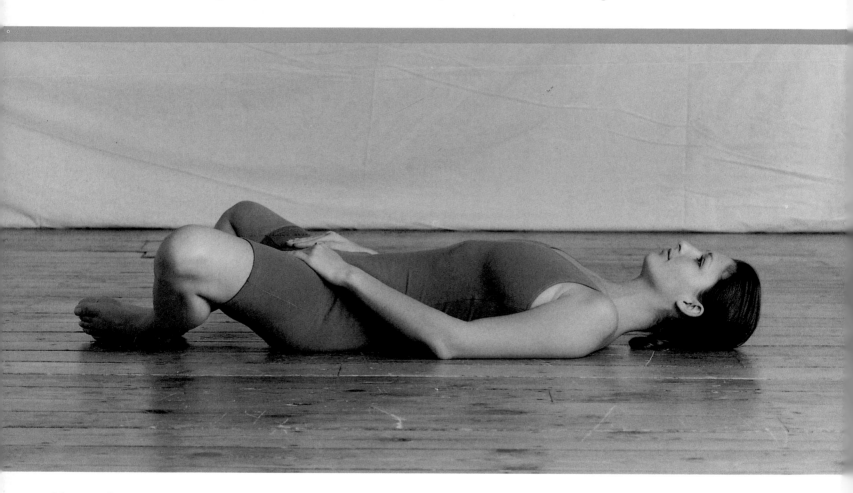

Diamond

Lie on your back with your knees bent and the soles of your feet touching. Have your heels as close to your buttocks as is comfortable, and aim to bring your knees as close as you can to the floor. Your lower back does not have to be pressed into the floor, so allow it to curve naturally. You should feel a stretch along your inner thighs. To increase the stretch, use your hands to push down gently on your thighs. Hold the stretch for at least 20 seconds. You can also do this stretch while sitting.

❶

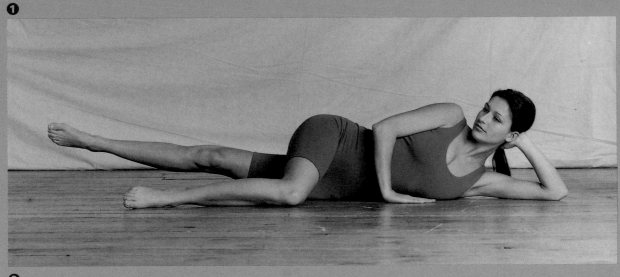

❷

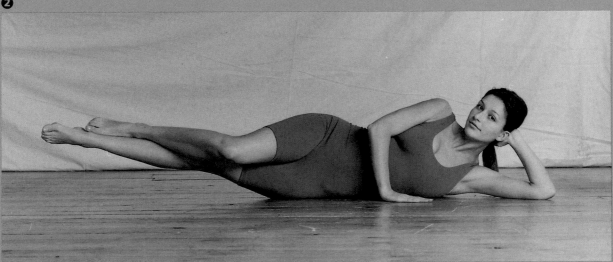

Lying lower leg lift

Lie on the floor on your left side with your legs stretched out, placing your right hand in front of your body to stabilize your torso, and rest your head on your left arm. Bend your right knee to a 90° angle and place it on the floor in front of you, so that your knee is in line with your hips. Lift your left leg, keeping it straight (1), and lower it until it nearly touches the floor before lifting it again. By keeping it slightly off the floor, you are maintaining tension in your leg, making the exercise more challenging. Breathe in as you lift your leg and out as you lower it, keeping the movements smooth and regular. Aim to repeat this around 20 times before resting and then switching sides.

For an advanced variation, rest your right leg on your left leg (2) so that as you lift your leg, you are working against the force of gravity with more of your body's weight.

❶

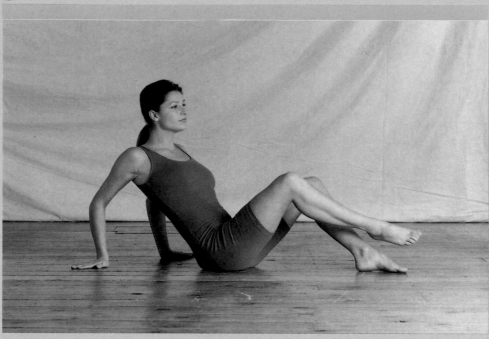

❷

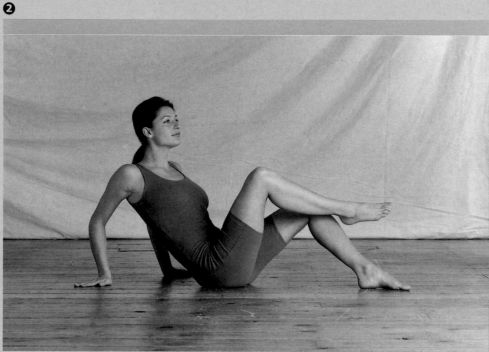

Seated leg hook

Sit on the floor, leaning back slightly with your knees bent, and place your hands behind you to stabilize your torso. Bring the heel of your right foot in front of the ankle of your left leg, and turn your right leg out so your inner thigh is almost facing the ceiling (1). Keeping a distance of an inch (2.5cm) between heel and shin, lift and lower your right heel up and down the length of your left shin (2).

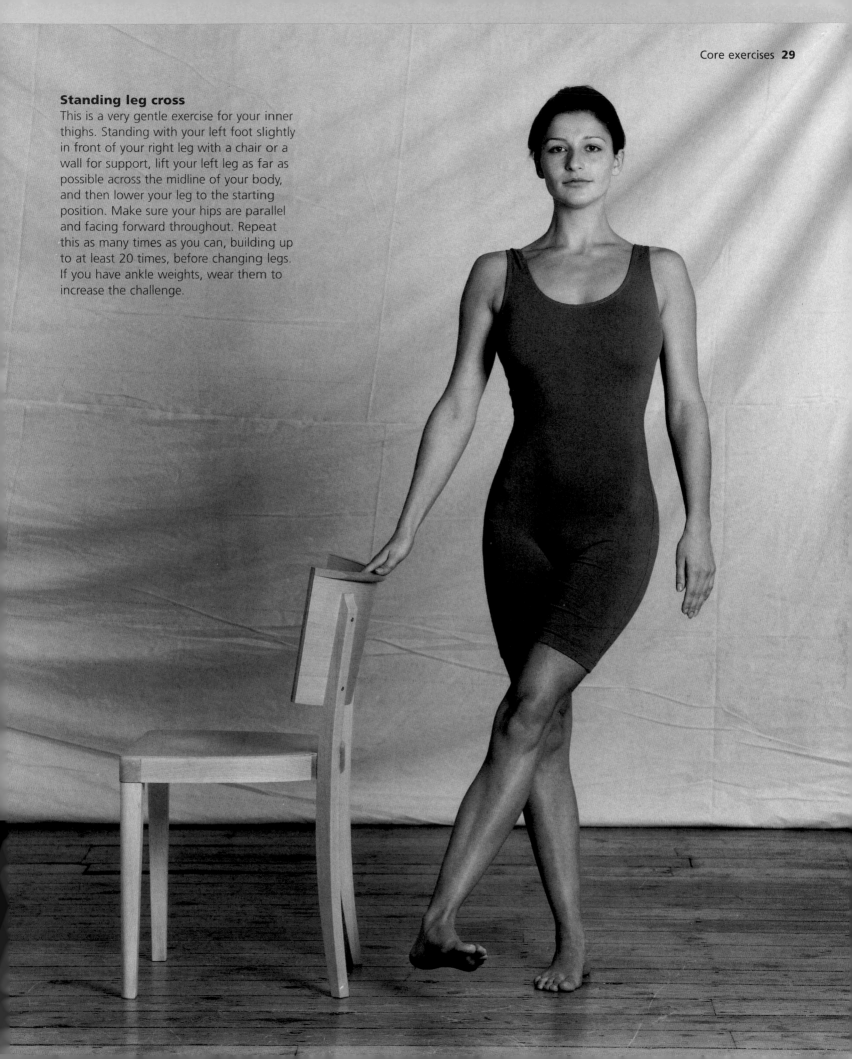

Standing leg cross

This is a very gentle exercise for your inner thighs. Standing with your left foot slightly in front of your right leg with a chair or a wall for support, lift your left leg as far as possible across the midline of your body, and then lower your leg to the starting position. Make sure your hips are parallel and facing forward throughout. Repeat this as many times as you can, building up to at least 20 times, before changing legs. If you have ankle weights, wear them to increase the challenge.

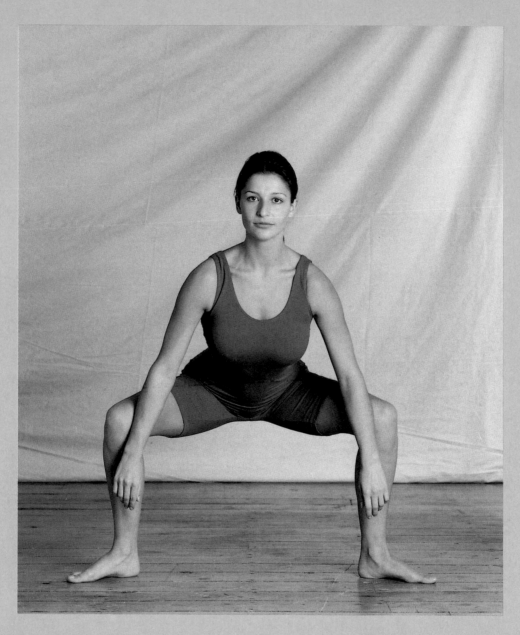

Plié press back

Standing with your feet a little more than shoulders' distance apart, turn your feet out, keeping your knees directly over your ankles and your knees and feet pointing in the same direction. Bend your knees, sticking your bottom out behind you, as you lower your hips almost to the level of your knees. Placing your forearms on the inside of your thighs, push gently against your thighs to increase the stretch. Make sure that your back is straight, your chest is lifted, and your abdominal muscles are pulled in. Hold this stretch for around 20 seconds, then straighten up and relax.

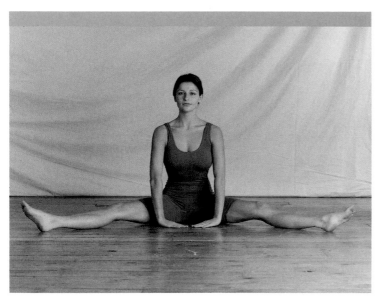

Wide V Stretch

Sitting on the floor with your legs straight out in front of you, move your legs apart until you feel an inner thigh stretch. Support yourself by placing your hands on the floor in front of you. Maintaining a long, strong back and good posture, lean forward slightly from the hips if you want to increase the stretch.

If you find this difficult, you can use gravity to help. Lie on your back and bend your knees in toward your chest, then straighten your legs up toward the ceiling. Ease your legs apart until you feel a stretch. To increase the stretch, you can press down gently with your hands on your inner thighs.

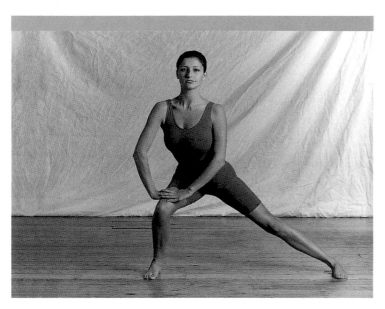

Side lunge

With your feet placed a little more than shoulders' width apart and slightly turned out, bend your right knee and shift your weight over to your right side. Try to keep your hips and chest facing forward, and check that your right knee is positioned over your ankle, your right knee and foot are facing in the same direction, and your left foot is flat on the floor. You can place your hands on the thigh of your bent leg for support, which will help you maintain the alignment of your upper body while you hold this stretch.

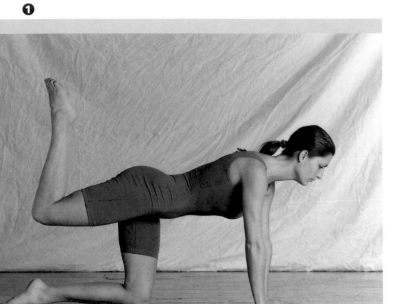

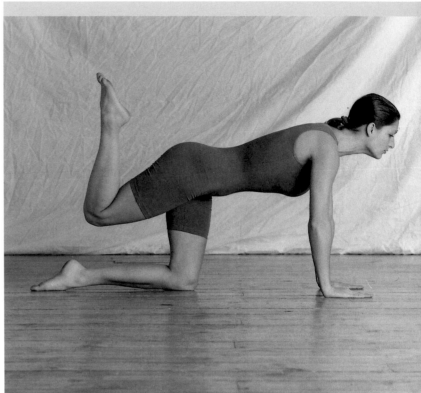

Kneeling knee cross-back

Kneel on all fours with your knees hips' distance apart. Place your forearms on the floor so your elbows are directly under your shoulders – when you are stronger, keep your arms straight. Raise your right leg straight out behind you, in line with your hip, and keeping your knee in line with your hip, bend it so your heel is toward the ceiling (1). Move your right knee across your left leg and down toward the floor (2), then lift your knee back in line with your hip. Repeat this 20 times before switching sides.

❶ 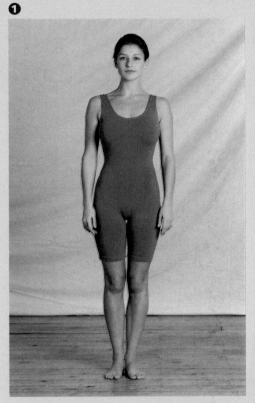 **❷** 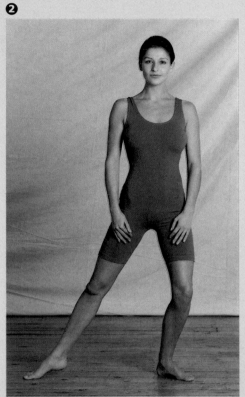 **❸**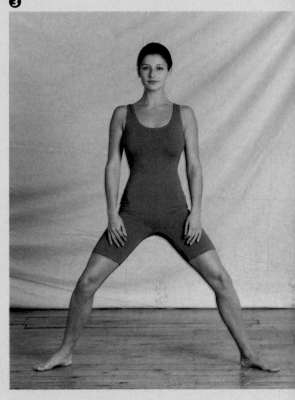

Slide

Stand with your feet together facing front (1), and step your right foot out to your right side so that your feet are at least shoulders' distance apart (2). Keeping your whole foot in contact with the floor and actually pushing your foot down on the floor, drag your right foot in toward your left foot (3) until your feet are together again. Make sure that your hips remain parallel and facing forward. Step out with your left foot and repeat on that side. Together these movements make one set.

The resistance you create by dragging your foot along the floor will make your inner thigh muscles work harder, but if you are doing this on carpet, beware of too much friction. Repeat as many times as you can, aiming for at least 20 sets.

Front thigh

The quadriceps, the muscle group located at the front of your thighs, work to straighten your knees, and they also help to protect your knees and the position of your knee caps. You must balance any strength work done on the quadriceps by also working on the hamstrings, the muscles at the back of your thighs (see pages 36–7).

You have to do most exercises for this muscle group in a standing position, unless you are working on specialized machines in a gym.

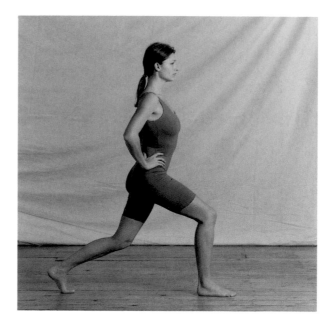

Forward lunge
Step forward two foot lengths with your right foot, and, at the same time, bend your left knee. Make sure that when you step forward, the knee of your front leg is over your ankle. If this is uncomfortable, you can shorten the distance you step forward.

❶

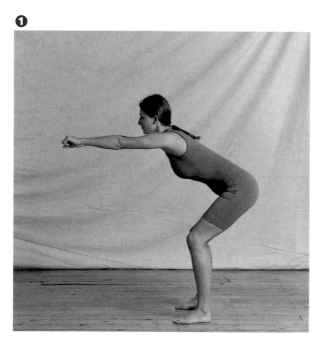

❷

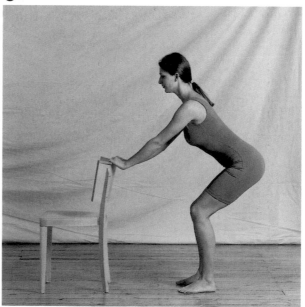

Parallel squat
Standing with your feet hips' width apart and your hands midway down your thighs for upper body support, bend your knees and slowly lower your hips down and back (but no lower than your knees) as you raise your arms until you look like a jockey on an imaginary horse. Your knees should remain above your ankles. Raise yourself upright just as slowly to a standing position. As you grow stronger, you can aim for the 20 repetition mark. To help balance, you can widen your stance slightly or hold on to a chair (2).

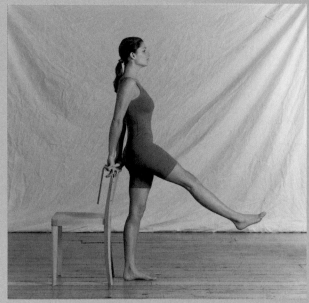

Standing leg raise

Using a chair or the wall for support, stand with your feet facing forward, a natural distance apart. Raise one leg in front of you, taking four beats to lift and the same to lower that leg. The slower the movement, the harder the muscles have to work. Repeat the action 20 times before changing legs.

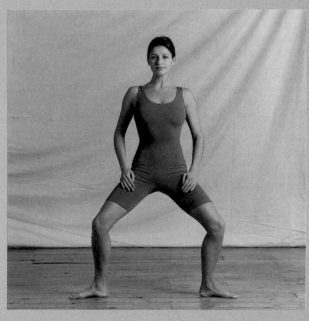

Plié squat

This is a variation of the parallel squat (opposite), with your hips open and your knees and feet turned out. Your knees should be in line with your ankles. This time, press your hips straight down and don't allow your bottom to stick out.

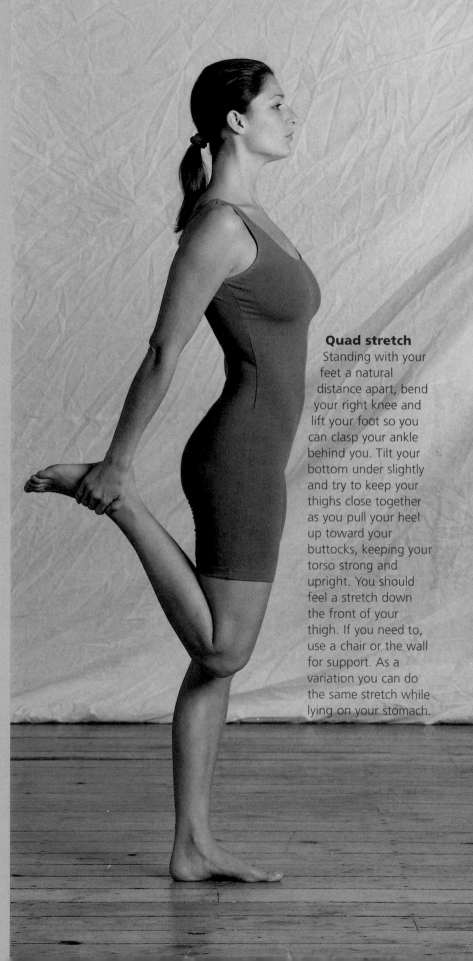

Quad stretch

Standing with your feet a natural distance apart, bend your right knee and lift your foot so you can clasp your ankle behind you. Tilt your bottom under slightly and try to keep your thighs close together as you pull your heel up toward your buttocks, keeping your torso strong and upright. You should feel a stretch down the front of your thigh. If you need to, use a chair or the wall for support. As a variation you can do the same stretch while lying on your stomach.

Rear thigh and buttocks

For most people, the hamstrings, at the rear of the thighs, are smaller and weaker than the quadriceps that oppose them, which makes them more susceptible to injury. You can address this imbalance with exercise. While most of the time you should do an equal number of exercises for the hamstrings and for the quadriceps, you can vary this occasionally by focusing more on the hamstrings – try doing a double set of hamstring curls after every set of front thigh exercises.

The muscles that make up your buttocks are known as the gluteus muscles, or gluts for short. With exercise, you can maintain and improve the firmness and shapeliness of your bottom. Other exercises to work these muscles are the parallel squat, the plié squat, and the forward lunge (see pages 34–5).

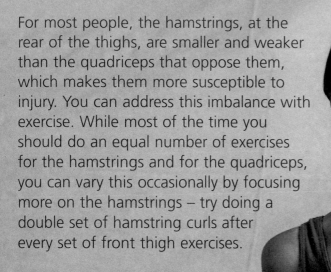

Seated crossover

Sit on the floor with your left leg on the floor and bent at the knee. Bend your right leg and cross it over your left leg, placing your right foot on the floor to your left. Keep your torso stabilized and your back tall as you place your left hand on the outside of your right knee and ease your knee over a little farther. Try to keep both buttocks on the floor. You will probably also feel this stretch along your outer thigh, and, if you gently twist and hold your body to look over your right shoulder, you should also feel a stretch in your lower back.

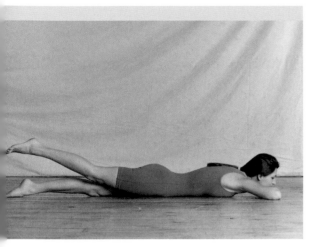 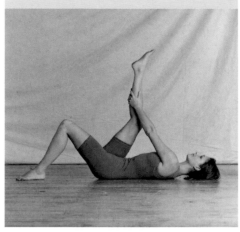 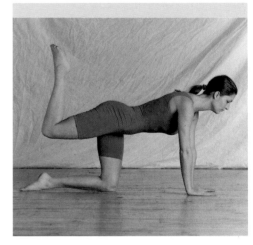

Rear leg lift

Lying face down on the floor (with your forehead resting on the back of your hands for comfort if you want), lift and lower your right leg as you keep both hipbones in contact with the floor. Focus on lifting from the top of your thigh while gently pressing your hips into the floor. If you are doing the exercise correctly, you will only be able to raise your leg a few inches off the floor. Each movement should be done in two to four beats. To make it easier, you can bend the knee of your lifting leg. Repeat the movement as many times as you can, aiming for 20 repetitions on each leg.

As an advanced variation, you can lift both legs at the same time, but great movement control is essential to protect your lower back.

Lying hamstring stretch

Lying on your back with your knees bent and your feet on the floor, pull your right thigh in toward your chest and aim to straighten your leg. Hold your thigh or your calf to support your leg.

To increase the stretch, pull gently on your leg to ease it closer to your chest. Remember, the stretch should be held for at least 20 seconds.

Hamstring curl

On all fours with your knees about hips' width apart – you should rest your forearms on the floor at first to stabilize your torso – raise your right leg straight out behind you so that your knee is aligned with your hip. Bend your knee to move your heel toward your buttocks, then straighten your leg out again. The timing of the movement should be moderate to slow, taking two to four beats to bring your heel in and the same to straighten your leg. Keep your torso stabilized and your head and neck aligned with your spine. When you have the strength in the torso to maintain good posture and your back does not sag, you can do the same exercise with straight arms, making sure that you do not lock your elbows.

Hip flexors and hip rotators

Your hip flexors are generally strong because they are used whenever you bend your knees to step up, and when you bend at the hip – to sit down, for example. Tight hip flexors can cause your bottom to protrude slightly, and your back may arch as the upper body is pulled forward, causing discomfort. You can address any imbalances between strength and flexibility by doing the stretch without the strength exercise once in a while.

Your hip rotators will usually be exercised while you work other muscle groups, and they do not normally need specific attention. However, you might want to focus on them occasionally.

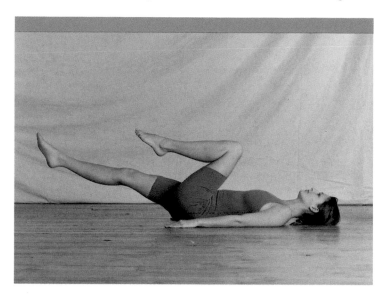

Leg extensions
Lying on the floor, bend your legs so that your knees are directly above your hips. Keeping your whole back on the floor, especially your lower back, straighten your right leg, then pull your right leg in as you extend your left leg. The motion is not cycling or circular, but a straight pressing out of your heel and a pulling in of your knee, done slowly and evenly, as if you were standing and alternately lifting your knees. Repeat the movement as many times as possible, aiming for at least 20 repetitions.

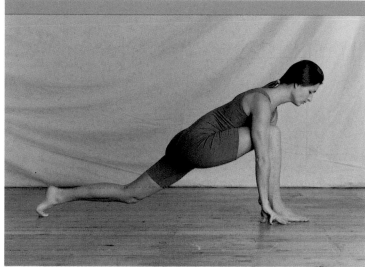

Low lunge
From a kneeling position, step your right foot forward, keeping your knee above your ankle and supporting yourself by placing your hands on the floor at either side of your right foot. Straighten your left leg behind you, keeping your toes on the floor, so you feel a stretch at the front of your hip and down the front of your thigh. Make sure you keep a straight line from your ear down to your hip. If you want to increase the stretch, you can bend your left knee slightly.

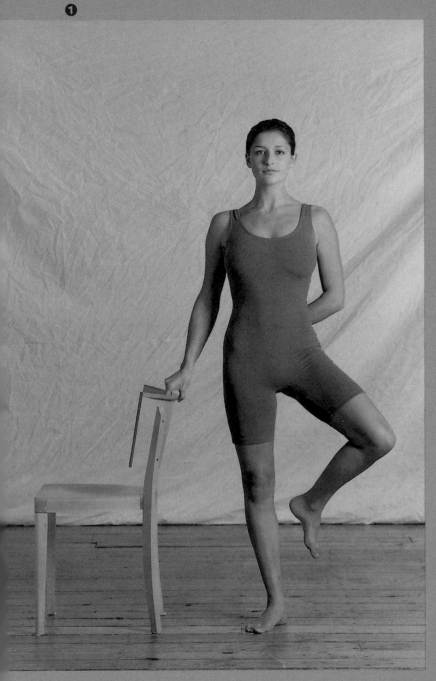

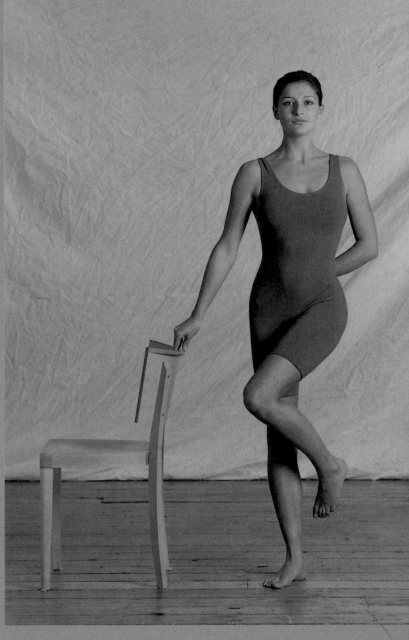

Standing hip rotation

Using a chair or a wall for support, balance on your right leg and bend your left leg at the knee and the hip. Lift your left knee up and across toward the right, then turn your leg out from the hip, moving your knee away from your body (1), then lift your left knee up and across to the right (2), in one flowing movement. Repeat at least 20 times, keeping the movement slow and even.

Warm-ups and cool-downs

Warm-up exercises create several responses in your body. In general, they make you more mentally alert and bodily aware. More specifically, they will gently mobilize your joints, lubricating them and preparing them for activity. Your respiration will increase, so there is more oxygen available for your working muscles. Your heart rate will also increase, speeding the movement of oxygen-carrying blood around your body. Your nervous system becomes more sensitive during a warm-up, so nerve impulses or messages are sent from brain to muscle more rapidly.

The best time to work on gentle stretching to improve your flexibility is during your cool-down, when your body is warm. At the same time, slower movements will bring your heart rate, body temperature, and respiration gradually back to a normal level.

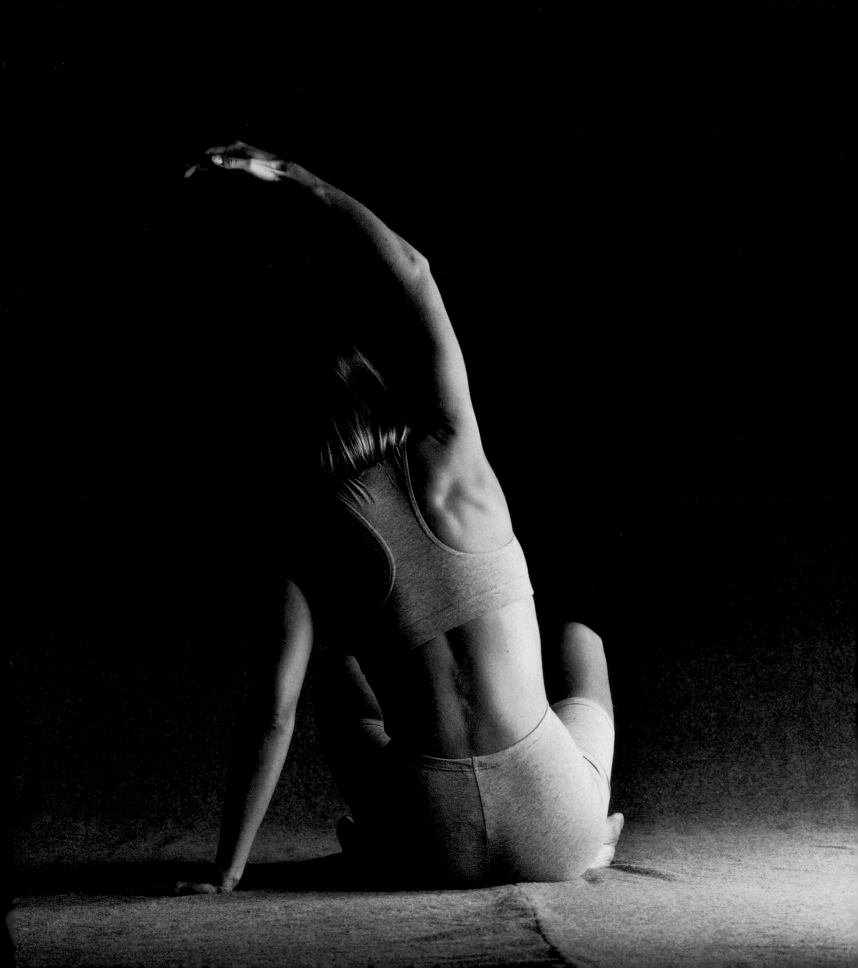

Warm-ups

Your warm-up should take eight to ten minutes, although if the room is cool or if you are feeling stiff or sluggish, take a little longer to make sure your body is properly prepared.

Make your movements as big as possible to take each joint through its full range of motion. Work at a pace that allows you to control all the movements and to flow one into the other. At first, changes from one move to another might be a little rough, but don't worry about this. As you become familiar with the exercises, they will start to flow – you can even put on some music to help your mood and pace. It is probably easier, in the beginning, to learn the leg and foot movements first, adding the arms once you are comfortable.

Finally, make sure everything you need for your exercise session is close by before you start your warm-up, so you will have fewer distractions and interruptions.

❶

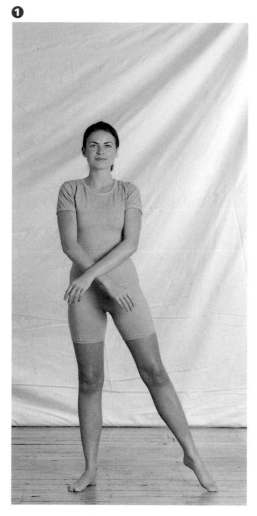

❷

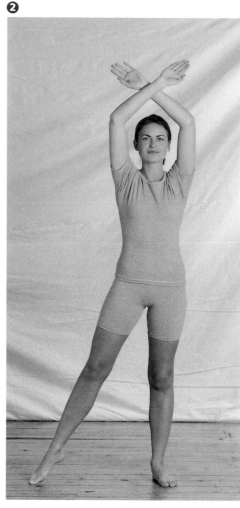

Press and heel lift

With your feet more than shoulders' width apart and slightly turned out, bend your knees, pressing both feet into the floor. Your weight should be balanced over both feet. As you straighten your legs, lift the heel of your left foot from the floor, transferring most of your weight onto your right leg and keeping your back straight. Return to the starting position by transferring your weight back over both feet, then repeat on the other side.

When you are comfortable, add the arm movements. You can roll your shoulders backward for eight counts, then change direction and roll them forward for eight counts (1). Once your shoulders have loosened up, try circling your arms in front of your body (2), then reverse the circles.

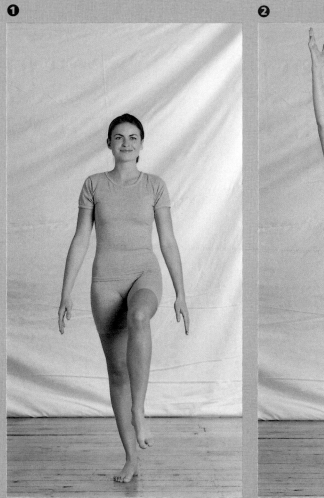

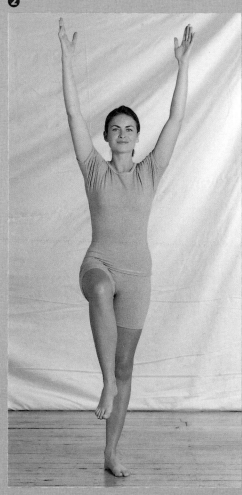

Stationary march

Maintaining good posture and alignment, gently march on the spot, staying light on your feet and letting your arms swing naturally by your side. March for 32 beats, moving back and forth if you want to. Once you establish your rhythm, you can add the arm movements. When your arms are down, exhale (1), then inhale as you raise them (2).

Pace yourself, synchronizing your feet and your breathing, taking four beats to inhale and four beats to exhale.

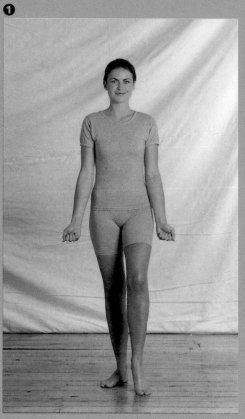

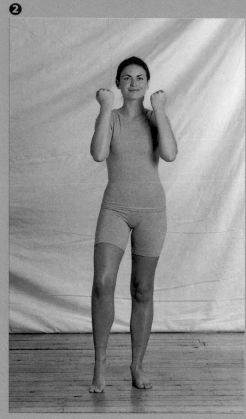

Touch and curl

Starting with your feet a little more than shoulders' width apart and slightly turned out, step your right foot in to your left foot, lightly touching the floor with your toe as your feet come together. Step out and forward with your right foot, placing your whole foot on the floor, and then step in with your left foot.

Repeat the movement from side to side, adding the arm movements. As you step to one side, straighten your arms, forming loose fists with your hands (1). As you step to the other side, bend your elbows so that your fists come up toward your shoulders, keeping your elbows fairly close to your waist (2).

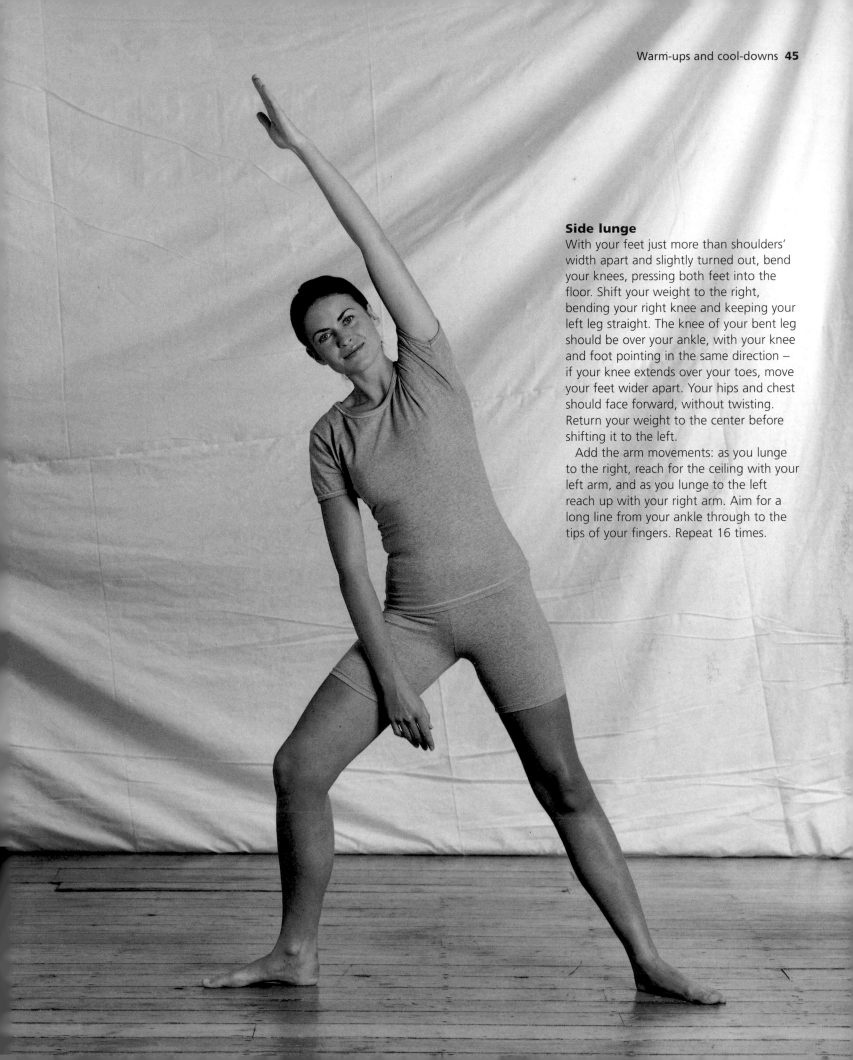

Side lunge

With your feet just more than shoulders'
width apart and slightly turned out, bend
your knees, pressing both feet into the
floor. Shift your weight to the right,
bending your right knee and keeping your
left leg straight. The knee of your bent leg
should be over your ankle, with your knee
and foot pointing in the same direction –
if your knee extends over your toes, move
your feet wider apart. Your hips and chest
should face forward, without twisting.
Return your weight to the center before
shifting it to the left.

Add the arm movements: as you lunge
to the right, reach for the ceiling with your
left arm, and as you lunge to the left
reach up with your right arm. Aim for a
long line from your ankle through to the
tips of your fingers. Repeat 16 times.

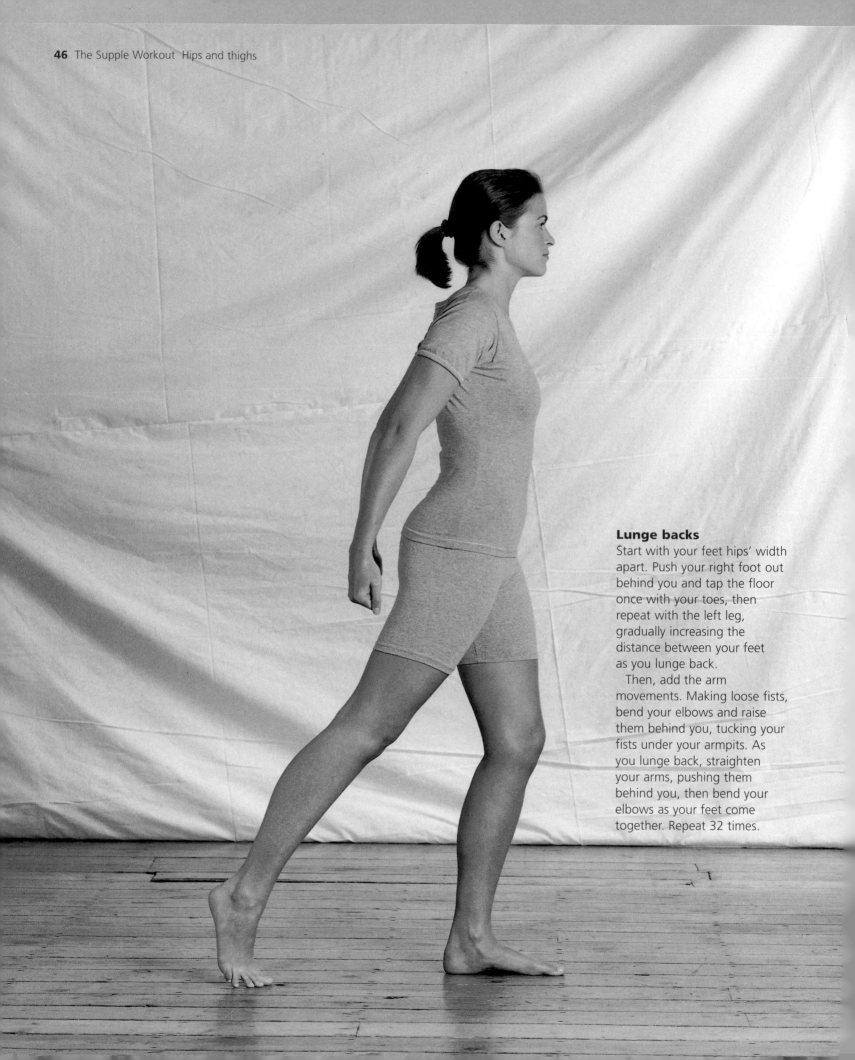

Lunge backs

Start with your feet hips' width apart. Push your right foot out behind you and tap the floor once with your toes, then repeat with the left leg, gradually increasing the distance between your feet as you lunge back.

Then, add the arm movements. Making loose fists, bend your elbows and raise them behind you, tucking your fists under your armpits. As you lunge back, straighten your arms, pushing them behind you, then bend your elbows as your feet come together. Repeat 32 times.

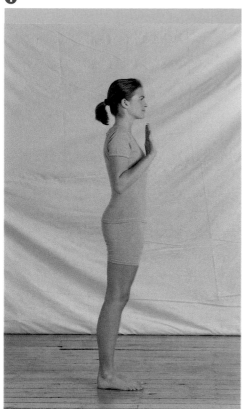

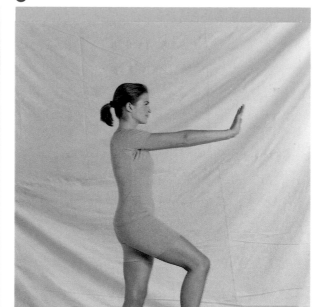

Knee lift and press

Starting with your feet a little more than shoulders' width apart and slightly turned out, shift your weight to the left, lifting your right knee slightly, keeping it lower than your hip.

Add the arm movements: bend your elbows at the side of your body, keeping them close to your chest, turning your palms out (1). When you lift your knee, extend your arms and push out with the palms of your hands (2). As you lower your knee, pull your arms back to your body. Repeat 16 times.

 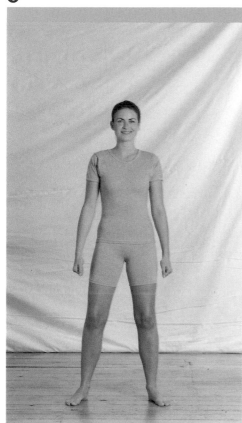

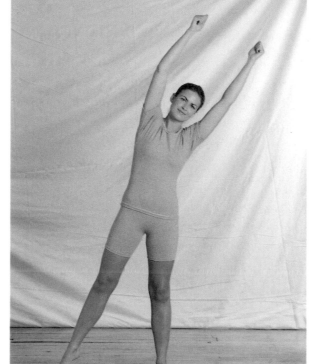

Side lift and punch

With your feet a little more than shoulders' width apart and slightly turned out, bend your knees slightly, pressing both feet into the floor. Your body weight should be balanced over both feet. As you straighten your legs, shift your weight to the left, raising your right leg out to the side, keeping your toes and hips facing forward.

Add your arms: as you bend your knees, punch toward the floor with your fists (1). As you straighten your legs, extend your arms high above your head and stretch to the side opposite your extended leg, breathing deeply (2). Repeat 16 times.

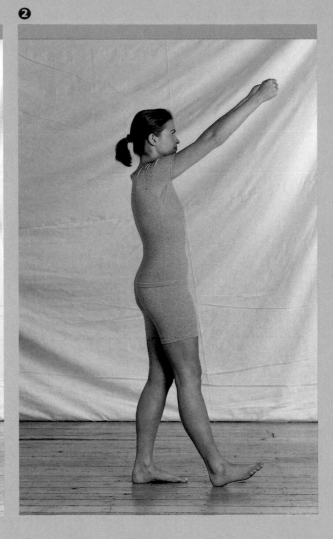

①

②

Dig and overhead press

Starting with your feet hips' width apart, move your right leg out in front, touching the floor with your heel and keeping your left knee slightly bent. Return your right foot to the starting position before stepping forward with the left.

Then add the arms: when your feet are together, rest your hands on your shoulders, with your elbows pointing out to the side (1). As you touch forward with your heel, raise your arms up (2). Repeat 16 times with synchronized arms and legs.

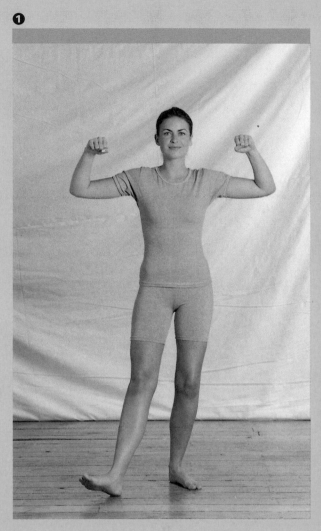

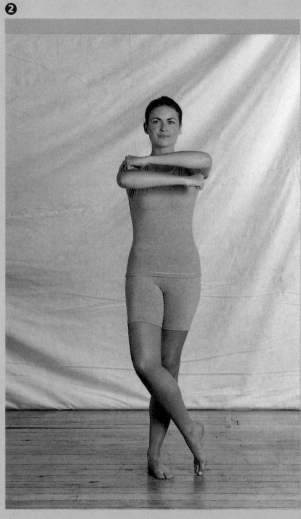

Heel-toe cross

Starting with your feet hips' width apart, move your right leg out in front and away from your body, so your heel touches the floor to your right, then bring that leg across your body and touch your toes to the floor to your left.

Once you are comfortable, add the arms: pull your elbows behind you to squeeze your shoulder blades together as you tap your heel (1). As you tap your toes, cross your arms in front of your chest (2). Repeat 16 times on each leg.

Cool-downs

A cool-down can take between 10 and 15 minutes out of every hour's exercise. As a general guideline, the more rigorous your exercise session, the longer your cool-down should be. Begin with the same type of movements you used in the warm-up, done at a much slower pace, then move on to stretches.

Finish with some conscious breathing. A few deep breaths as you stand and stretch as tall as you can will leave you feeling strong and vibrant, and a longer spell of floor relaxation, enjoying deep breathing, will make you feel peaceful and luxurious.

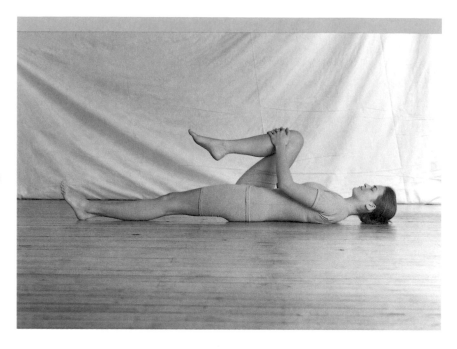

Hip flexor stretch
Lying on your back, bring your right knee to your chest, clasping it lightly. Gently press your left leg to the floor as you pull your right knee closer to your chest. Hold for 30 seconds before repeating with the other leg.

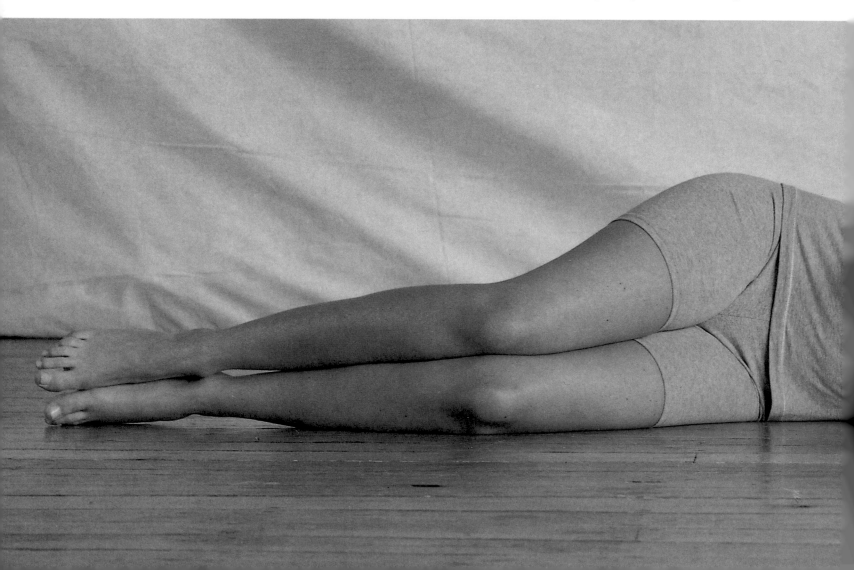

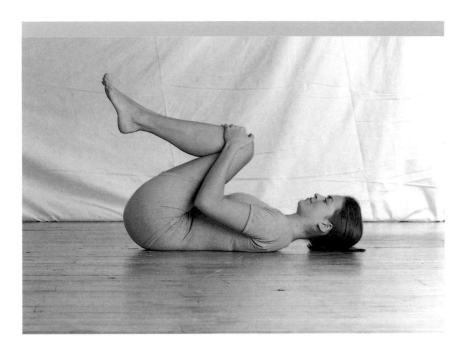

Lower back stretch

Lying on your back, keeping your neck long, hug your knees toward your chest. Your hips will rise slightly off the floor. Hold this position for around 30 seconds before lowering your legs slowly to the floor.

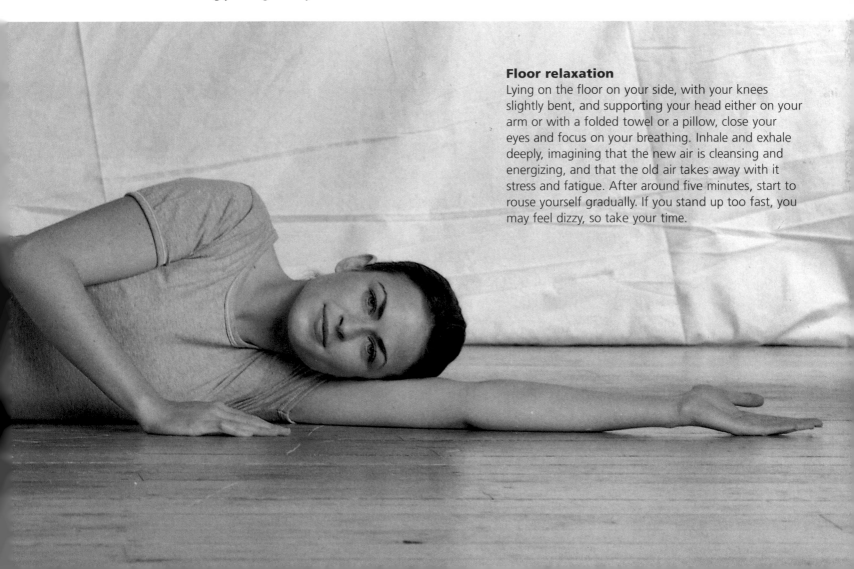

Floor relaxation

Lying on the floor on your side, with your knees slightly bent, and supporting your head either on your arm or with a folded towel or a pillow, close your eyes and focus on your breathing. Inhale and exhale deeply, imagining that the new air is cleansing and energizing, and that the old air takes away with it stress and fatigue. After around five minutes, start to rouse yourself gradually. If you stand up too fast, you may feel dizzy, so take your time.

Total body workout

When you are targeting hips and thighs in your exercise routines, it is important not to neglect the other parts of your body. Otherwise, you could cause muscular imbalances that increase the risk of injury. It is worth paying particular attention to the upper body, because women, in particular, are often comparatively weak in that area. Try to vary your exercise pattern, alternating one session where you focus exclusively on your hips and thighs with another where you can take a more holistic approach.

Although sometimes more than one exercise is presented here for a particular part of the body, choose only one or two exercises and put as much effort into those as possible. Begin by doing as many repetitions as you can, aiming, as you get stronger, for 20 without resting, and trying to hold all stretches for around 20 to 30 seconds.

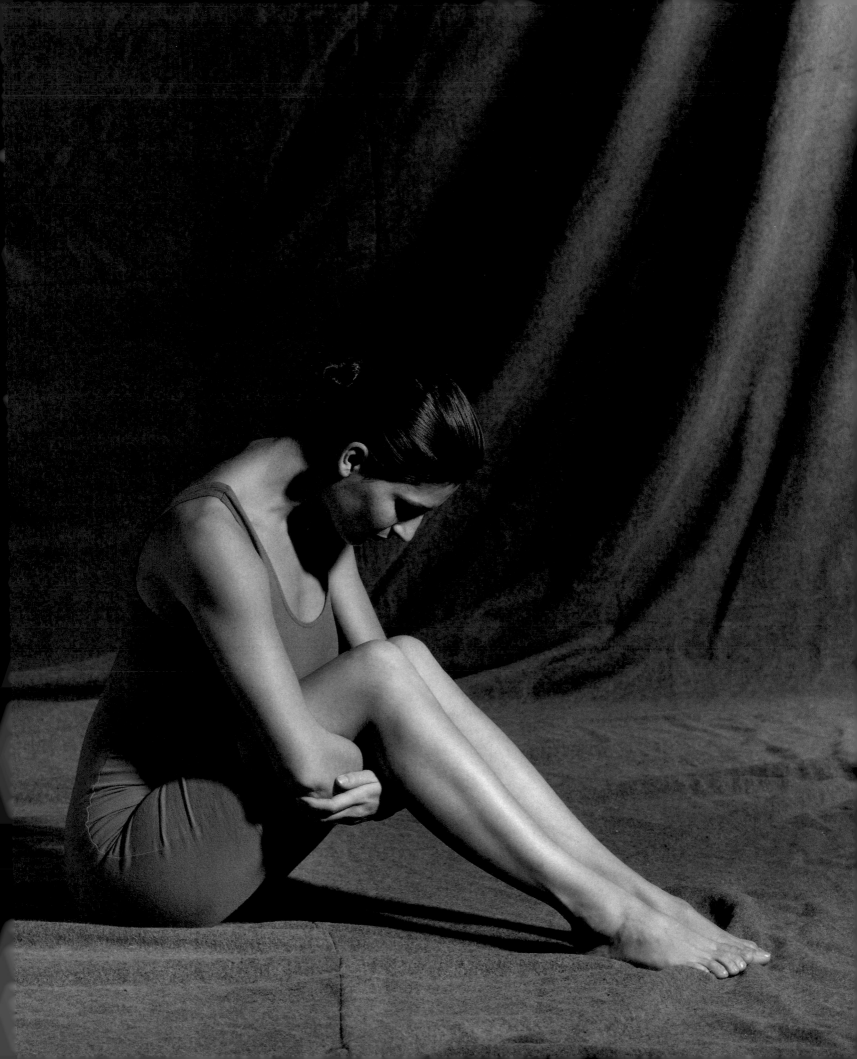

Shoulders and upper body

The muscles of your shoulders, the deltoids, are small, particularly compared to your buttocks and thighs, so they may tire easily when you first start exercising and later if you start to use weights.

Don't worry about this – rest between repetitions and ease your shoulders out with shoulder rolls and other gentle stretches. If you are suffering from stress, these stretches can also help you to relax.

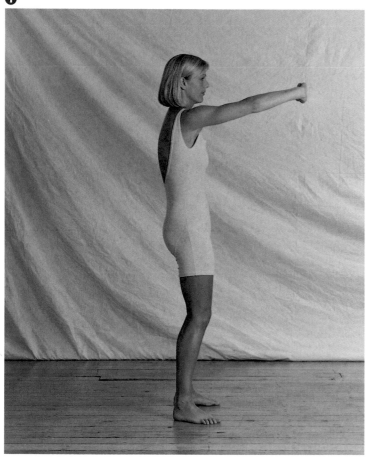

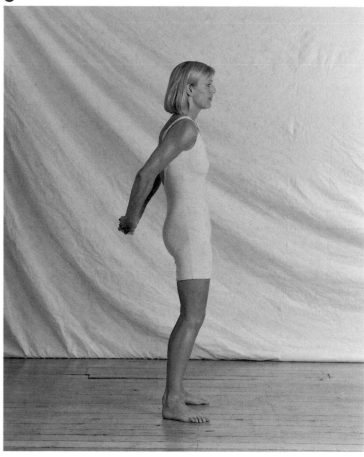

Upper body stretch

Bring your arms in front of you and link your fingers. Turn your palms out to face front and push away with your hands as you straighten your arms (1). Your back should be rounded and your shoulders rolled in as you stretch the back of your body. Then clasp your hands behind your back and raise your arms up and away from your body to stretch your front (2).

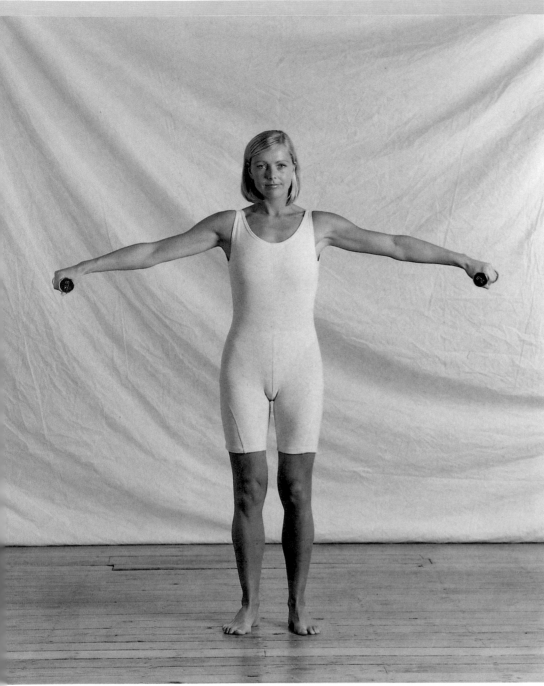

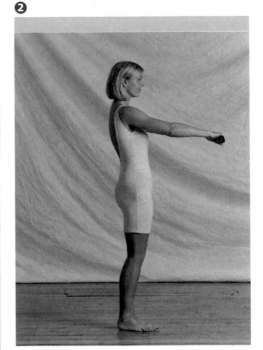

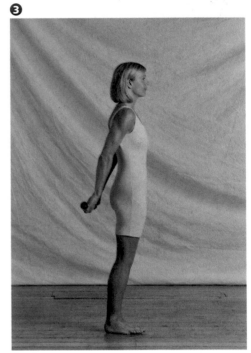

Raise and press

Each stage of this exercise will work a different area of your shoulder muscles.

Begin standing with good posture. For the middle of your shoulders, start with your arms by your side and your palms turned in toward your thighs. Raise your arms out to the side, no higher than shoulder level (1), then lower them.

For the front of your shoulders, start with your arms by your side and your palms facing back. Slowly lift your arms out in front of you to the level of your shoulders, keeping your palms facing down (2), then, just as slowly, lower them.

The last variation targets the back of your shoulders. Place your arms behind your back, resting the back of your hands on your buttocks. Slowly raise your arms behind you as far as they will go (3), and then gradually lower your arms back to the starting position. Make sure that your torso remains stable and upright and that you do not lean forward or roll your shoulders as you raise your arms.

To enhance any of these exercises, you can use weights, increasing the size as you grow stronger.

Biceps and triceps

Working in opposition, the biceps and the triceps are the main muscles in the upper arms. The biceps allow you to lift your arms in front of you, bend your elbows, and turn your palms up and down. Because they are used so frequently, they are often stronger than other upper body muscles. In most people, they are also stronger than the triceps, which lower your arms and straighten your elbows.

When you exercise your arms, you want to aim for increased strength and balance. As your arms become stronger, many day-to-day tasks, from carrying bags to working at a computer, will become easier. As your triceps develop in line with your biceps, you will experience more ease and fluency in your movement.

❶

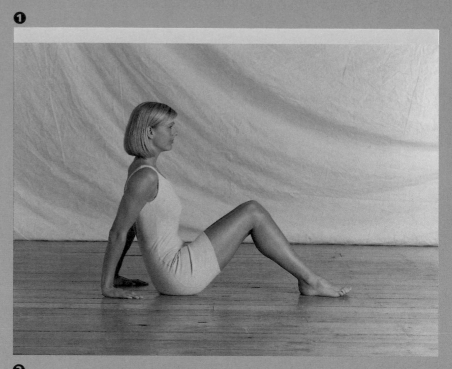

❷

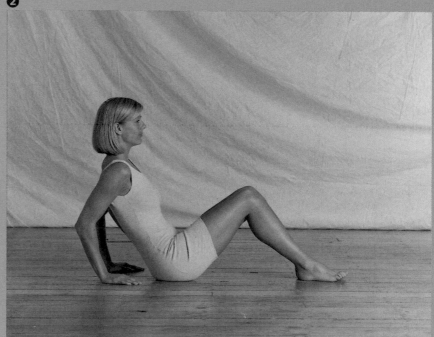

Tricep dips
This is the easiest version of the tricep dip. Begin by sitting on the floor with your knees bent and your feet flat on the floor. Place your hands on the floor behind you, shoulders' width apart, with your fingers facing forward: this will help you to stabilize your torso (1). By bending your elbows, ease your upper body halfway toward the floor (2), then straighten your arms, returning your upper body to the start position. Repeat 20 times.

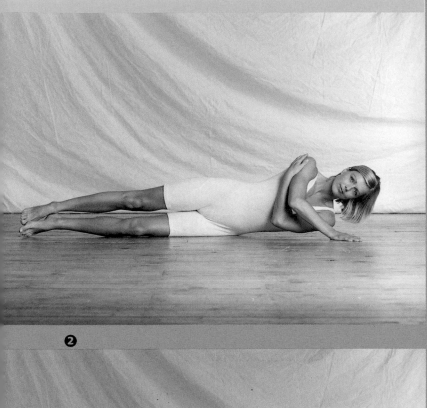

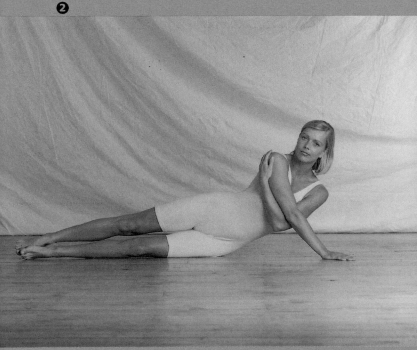

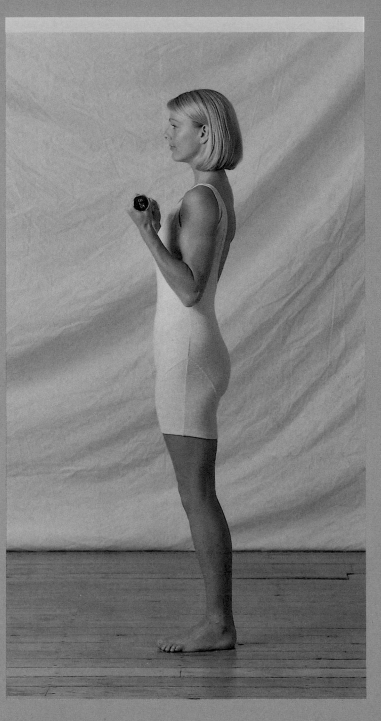

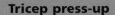

Tricep press-up

This is a very advanced exercise. Lie on your left side with both knees slightly bent, and place your right palm down on the floor in front of your chest for stability. Wrap your left arm under your right and place your left hand on top of your right shoulder (1). By pressing up with your right arm, raise your torso (2), then lower it by bending your elbow, making sure both movements are done slowly and with control. Stabilization is all-important in this exercise, so don't forget to pull in your abdominals and keep your back straight.

Bicep curl

Standing straight and strong, turn your palms away from you and make loose fists. Slowly bend your elbows and pull your forearm up to meet your biceps. Your wrists should be straight throughout. Gently lower your arms to the starting position before repeating 20 times. You can enhance this exercise by using weights, but make sure you do not rock your body as you raise and lower your arms. As a variation, you can turn your palms to face your thighs, and as you bend your elbows to raise your forearms, your thumbs head in toward your shoulders.

Upper back and lower back

Back pain, an all-too-common complaint these days, often results from weak back muscles and bad posture, particularly when sitting. The back muscles, working with the muscles of your chest and your abdomen, stabilize your torso and hold your body upright. Exercises that help to strengthen the back will help you to improve and maintain your posture and to avoid discomfort.

If you sit and stand with rounded shoulders, the muscles of your upper back are held in a continuously stretched position. In this case, you should emphasize exercises that strengthen this part of your body. It is in your lower back that you will feel the strain most.

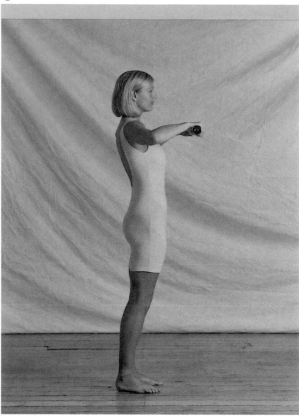

Standing fly

Standing with your feet hips' distance apart, bend your elbows and raise them out to the sides in line with or just forward of your shoulders and just slightly lower than your shoulders (1). Pull your elbows behind your back as if you were trying to get them to touch (2). You should feel your shoulder blades squeeze together. Gently release your shoulder blades, allowing your elbows to return to the starting position, and repeat 12 to 20 times. Make sure you maintain good posture throughout the movement.

  You can do the same movement more effectively by lying on the floor on your stomach, because you will be working against gravity. Without lifting your head, raise your elbows and pull them behind you, squeezing your shoulder blades together. Release and lower them to the floor, before repeating up to 20 times.

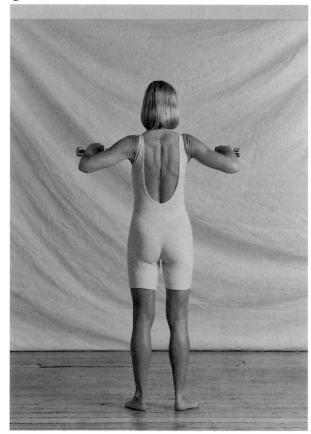

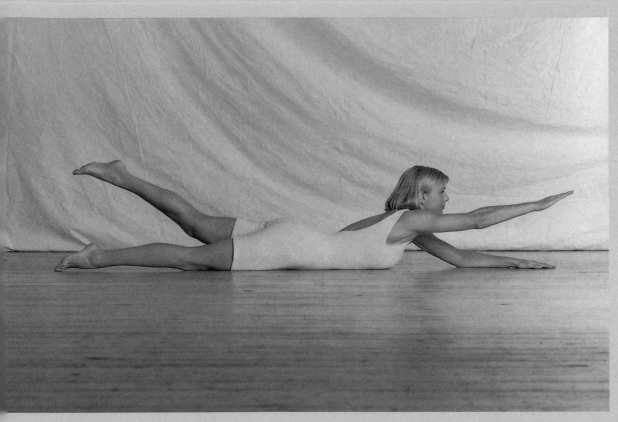

Opposite arm and leg lift

Lie on your stomach with your arms stretched out above your head. Keeping your hips and chest on the floor, lift your right arm and your left leg at the same time to the same height. Hold for as long as you are comfortable, aiming for 20 seconds. Lower the arm and leg to the floor, before repeating with your left arm and right leg.

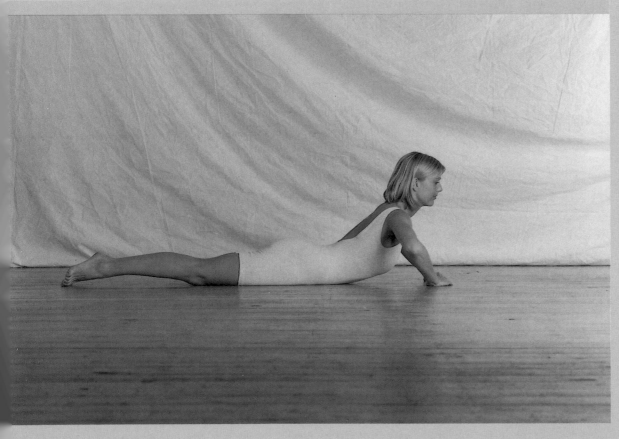

Lower back extension

Lying on your stomach with your hands under your chin, keep your hipbones and your feet on the floor as you press through your arms and lift your upper body off the floor as if it were one solid unit: visualize your spine as a metal rod that extends through your neck to the top of your head, so your head remains in a natural position. Although you should feel a pull along your back, you should not feel any discomfort. Use your arms for support as you lower your body back to the floor.

As an advanced variation, you can place your hands lightly on the small of your back or on your buttocks.

Chest

Much of our day-to-day movement is done to the front of our bodies. Think about the actions involved in pushing a shopping cart, working at a computer, or picking up an object from the floor or from a table.

To counteract the effects of the dominance of the front of the body, it is important to stretch out the chest muscles. At the same time, a strong and supple chest area helps to promote good posture, because it will prevent the shoulders from rolling

and the upper back from rounding both during exercise and other activity and at rest.

Since the front of the body tends to be stronger than the back, any exercises done for the chest should be complemented by upper back exercises (see page 58–9) to develop a balanced torso.

As always, begin by working gently, especially if you have not done much work on your chest and upper back in the past.

❶

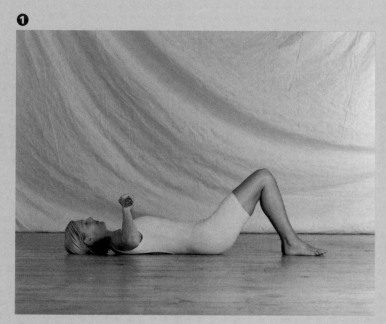

❷

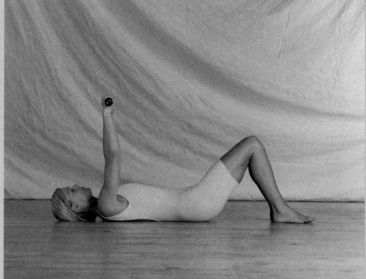

Chest press

Lie on your back with your arms straight out to the side, your knees bent, and your feet on the floor, and bend your elbows so your knuckles face the ceiling, trying to keep your upper arms in contact with the floor (1). Raise your elbows off the floor and

straighten your arms toward the ceiling (2), then gently lower your arms, bending your elbows until they are again in contact with the floor. With practice, you can add weights to this exercise, increasing their size as you grow stronger.

❶

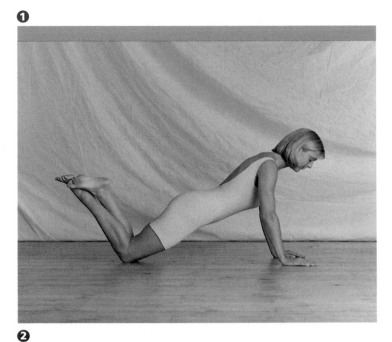

❷

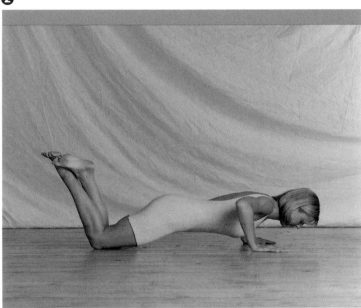

Press-up

On all fours, with your knees hips' width apart and your arms shoulders' width apart, lift your feet, cross your ankles, and lean forward, creating a straight line of your body from your knees to your ears (1). This line should be held as you slowly lower your body toward the floor by bending your elbows (2), then raise it slowly as you straighten them.

   If you find this difficult, you can try the "box" press-up. Kneel on all fours, keeping your hips over your knees and your shoulders over your elbows and wrists. Bend your elbows and lower your chest toward the floor. Your nose is likely to touch the floor before your chest does. Stabilize your torso so your lower back does not sag, and keep your neck in alignment with your spine.

Torso

These gentle stretches will complement the strength moves you have done to work your upper and lower back, your chest, and your abdominals.

Strength exercises involve repeated contractions of the muscles. This means that they can cause the muscles to shorten, but complementary stretches will reverse that effect. They will help you to remain supple even as you are becoming stronger. Gently stretching your muscles after exertion will also help you to relax before moving to the next stage.

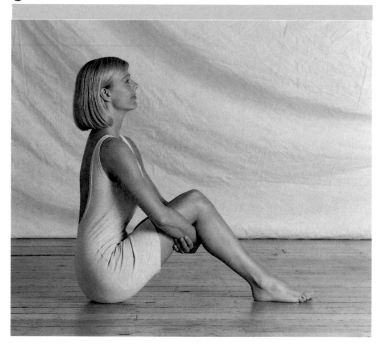

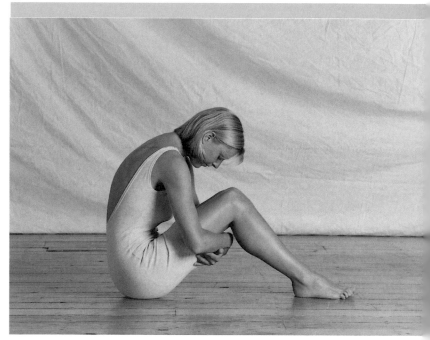

Crossed-arm back stretch
Sit on the floor with your knees bent and your feet on the floor. Wrap your arms under your knees, clasping your elbows (1). As you pull your abdominals in, lift and expand your back by separating your shoulder blades (2). Keep your arms clasped, using the resistance to enhance the stretch. Hold this stretch for around 20 seconds, then release and relax.

❶

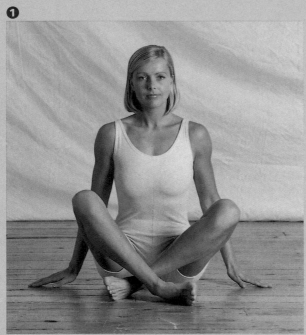

Sitting torso stretch

Sitting on the floor cross-legged, or in any other comfortable position (1), place your right hand on the floor to your right side for support, and reach your left arm overhead, feeling the stretch down the left side of your body (2). Hold this stretch for 20 seconds before relaxing, then switching sides.

❷

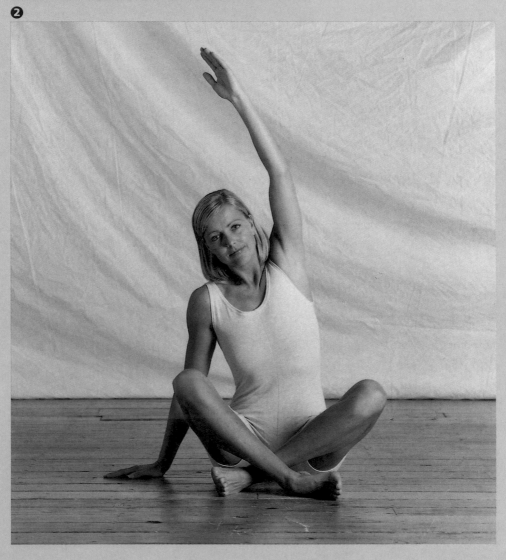

Abdominals

These types of abdominal exercise work the muscles safely but intensively. When you begin, do as many repetitions as you can manage, but remember, you are aiming for at least 20.

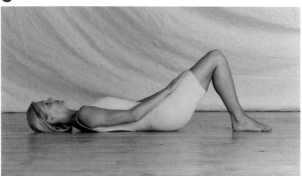

Curl-up

Lie on your back with your knees bent and your feet on the floor. Place your hands on your thighs (1). Pull your stomach muscles to close the gap between your back and the floor, then contract your stomach muscles so that your upper back, shoulders, and head lift (2). With control, lower your upper body toward the floor and, just before you get to a position where you feel you can relax, immediately repeat the sequence. Your chin should be in a natural position.

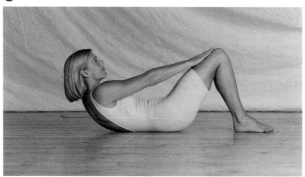

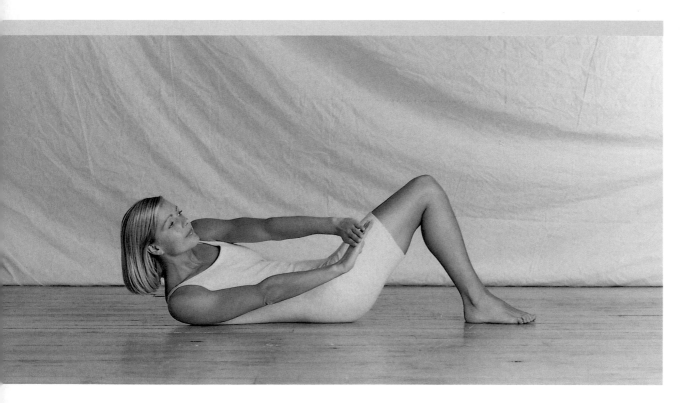

Oblique curl

This exercise is similar to the curl-up, but as you contract your abdominals, lift your left shoulder up and over toward your right hip, keeping your right shoulder on the floor. Slowly release your abdominals to lower your left shoulder to the floor. Your head and neck should remain in a natural position throughout. As a variation, you can place your right heel on your left thigh, and as you contract your abdominals, you should lift your left shoulder over toward your right knee.

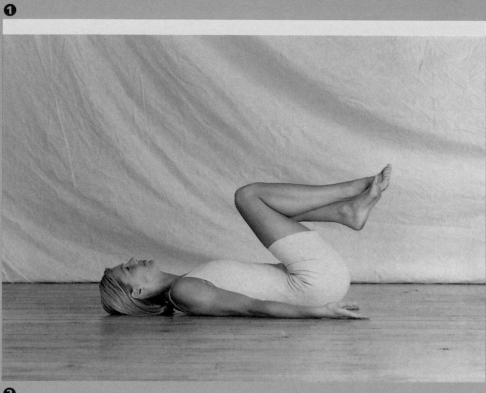

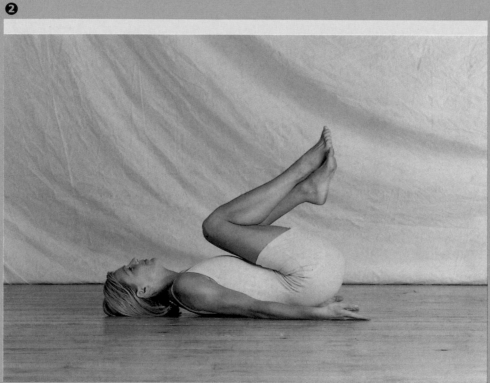

Reverse curl

Lying on your back with your arms by your side and your palms turned up, bring both knees toward your chest, allowing your lower back to press into the floor. Cross your ankles and keep your heels close to your buttocks (1). As you contract your abdominals, your hips will lift up and forward and your knees will move toward your shoulders (2). Release in a slow, controlled manner, and repeat.

Legs

When exercising, it is easy to forget your lower legs, ankles, and feet. But wearing restrictive shoes can make this area of your body very tense and tight, so it is important to stretch from time to time. Also, the muscles in this region absorb a lot of the stress of walking, jumping, and running, and they will be more resilient when they are stronger and more supple.

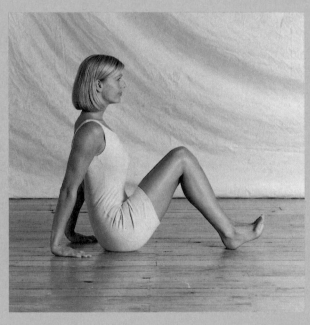

Toe taps
Sitting with bent knees and feet on the floor, lift and lower your toes and feet in a slow toe tap, keeping your heels on the floor. You can either work both feet at once, or alternate from right to left with single lifts. If you turn your feet in and out as you tap, you will be working with the muscles that run down the side of your legs to your ankles.

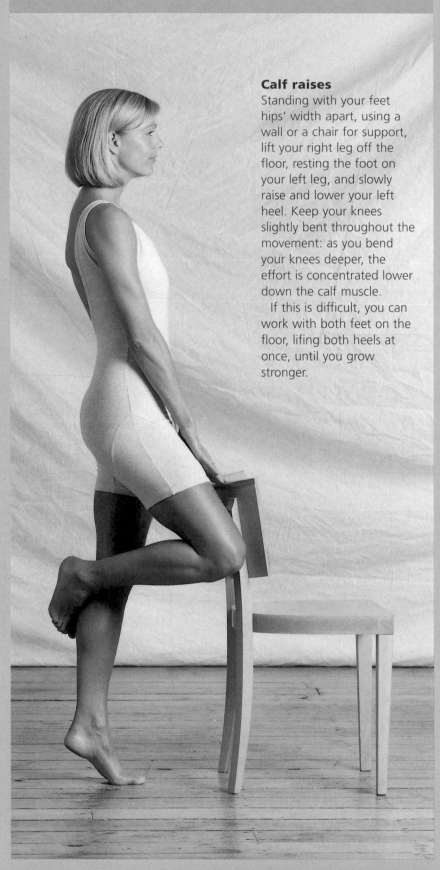

Calf raises
Standing with your feet hips' width apart, using a wall or a chair for support, lift your right leg off the floor, resting the foot on your left leg, and slowly raise and lower your left heel. Keep your knees slightly bent throughout the movement: as you bend your knees deeper, the effort is concentrated lower down the calf muscle.

If this is difficult, you can work with both feet on the floor, lifing both heels at once, until you grow stronger.

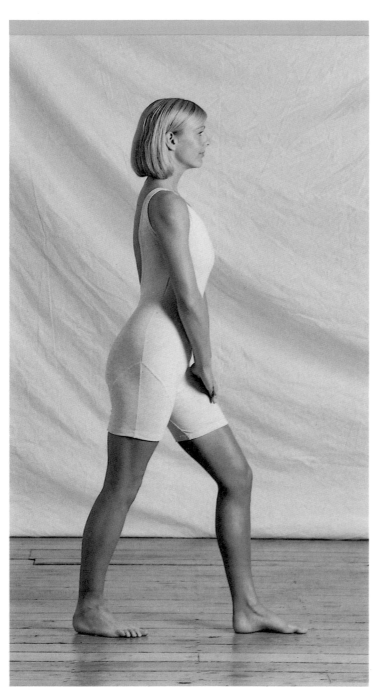

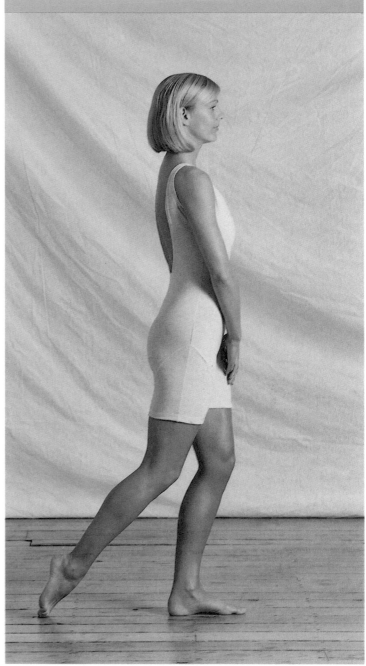

Calf stretch

Stand in a lunge position, with one foot in front of the other, and the knee of your front leg slightly bent and directly over your ankle. Move your rear leg farther back, keeping the heel of that foot on the floor, until you feel a stretch in your calf muscle. Hold for 30 seconds before repeating on the other leg.

If you bend the knee of your rear leg slightly, still keeping your heel on the floor, stepping in with your rear leg if you need to, you will feel a deeper stretch that works your lower calf.

Shin stretch

In a lunge position, lift your back foot and turn it under so the tops of your toes are resting on the floor. Bend the knee of your back leg and press the top of your foot toward the floor. You will feel the stretch along the top of your foot and in your shin. Hold for up to 30 seconds, then repeat on the other leg.

Routines

To save time and challenge yourself further, you can combine different exercises to devise a comprehensive workout covering your entire body. If you add together a hamstring curl and a tricep press-up, for example, you will be involving your whole body in dynamic movement.

By changing the combinations from time to time, you add variety to your exercise sessions. Think about changing your exercise routine every four to six weeks to keep yourself motivated – or you can have two different workouts that you alternate.

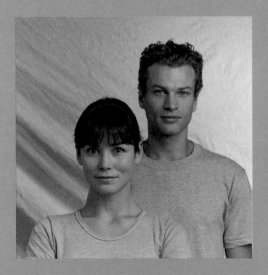

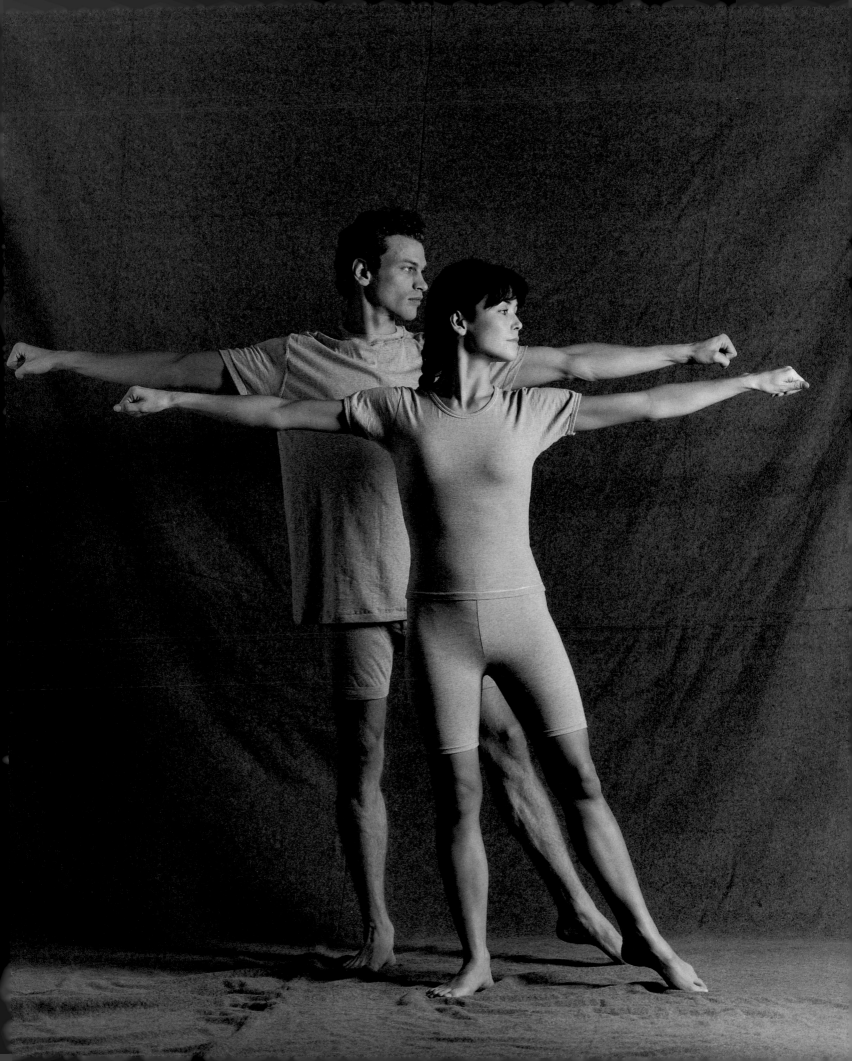

❶

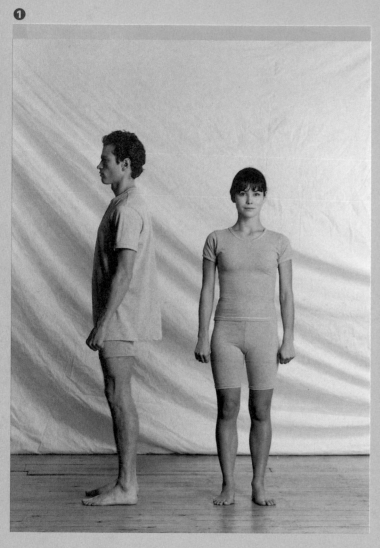

❷

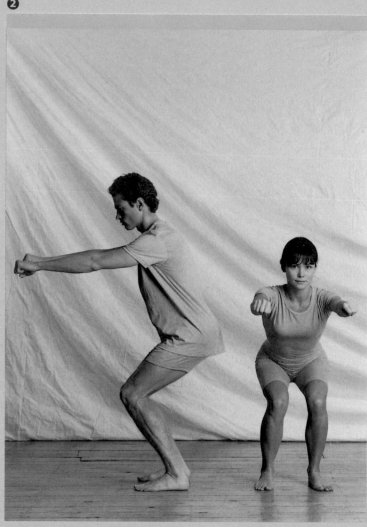

Squat and raise

Standing with your feet hips' width apart (1), bend your knees slowly to bring your hips down and back but no lower than your knees. As you squat, raise your arms out in front of you to shoulder height (2). The deeper you squat, the harder your legs will be working. As you stand up, lower your arms to your sides. Allow the movements to flow from one to the other.

If you want to make the exercise more challenging for your upper body, you can hold weights.

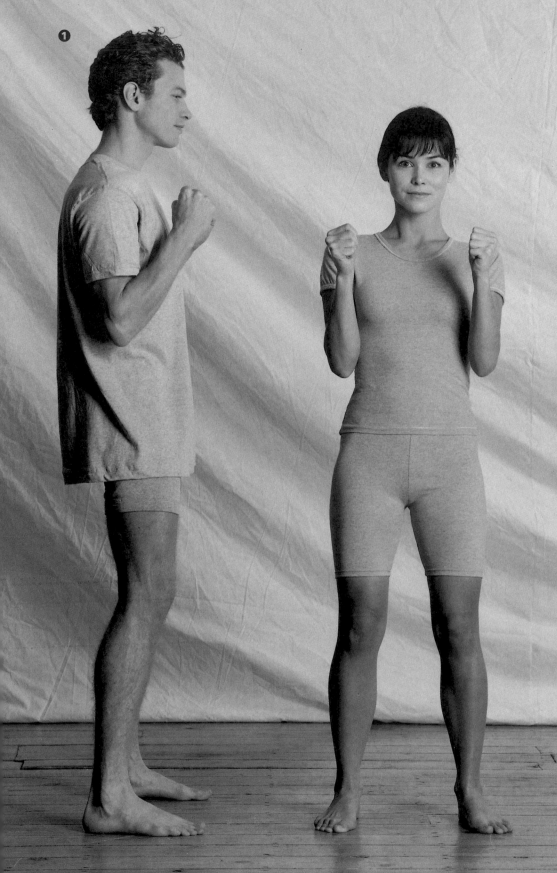

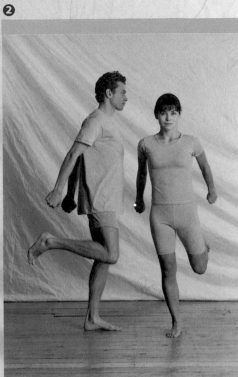

Tricep kickback

Begin with your feet wider than hips'
width apart, your elbows bent close to
your waist, and your hands in fists (1).
Shifting your weight onto your right foot,
lift your left foot behind you, like a
standing hamstring curl. At the same time,
straighten your elbows and push your
arms behind your body (2). Return to the
start and repeat on the other side.

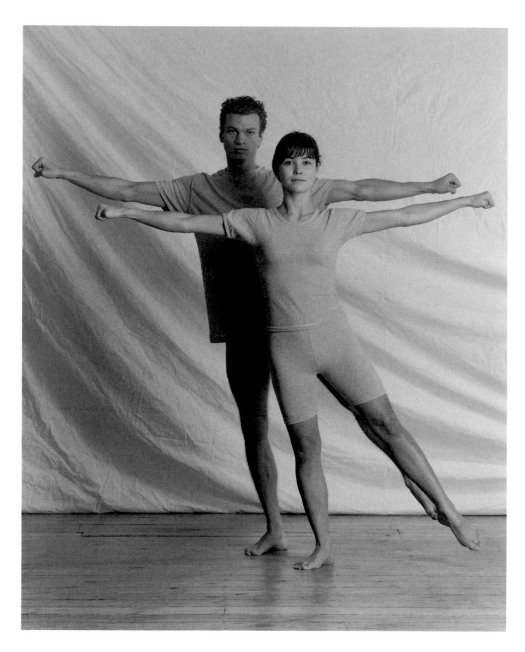

Arm and leg raise

Begin with your legs wider than hips' width apart and your knees bent. Straightening your right leg, raise your left leg out to the side at the same time as you raise both arms out to your sides to shoulder height. Return to the starting position, then repeat on the other side.

It is important to keep all the movements dynamic – when you return to the starting position, really punch your hands to the floor, and when you raise your leg to the side, make sure it is a strong movement. Work in a controlled fashion, making all your movements as big as you can.

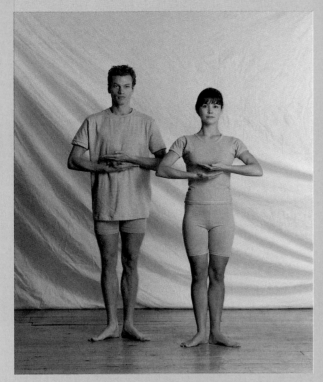

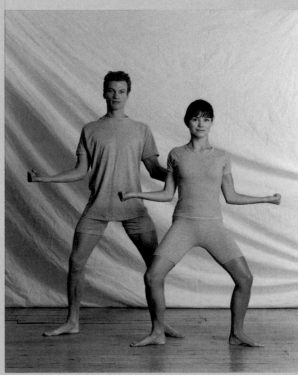

Cross and slide

Begin with your feet hips' width apart and slightly turned out, and your arms crossed in front of you (1). Step your legs apart to the left, bending your knees, at the same time as you open your arms, bringing your hands away from your body and your elbows in to contact with your waist (2). Slide your left foot back to the center, crossing your arms again.

You can increase the challenge in three ways: holding weights; making the squat deeper; and pressing your foot harder onto the floor as you slide.

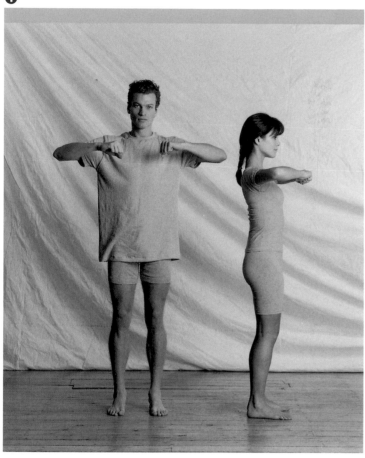 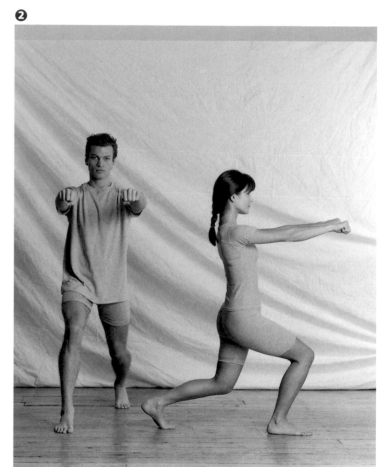

Chest press and forward lunge

Begin with your feet hips' width apart and your elbows bent and held out to the side at shoulder or chest level (1). As you step forward into a lunge, making sure you keep your front knee above your ankle, press your arms forward as if you were pushing something away (2). Bring your arms back toward your body as you step your feet back together.

You can challenge your muscles further by increasing the depth of your lunge or by holding weights.

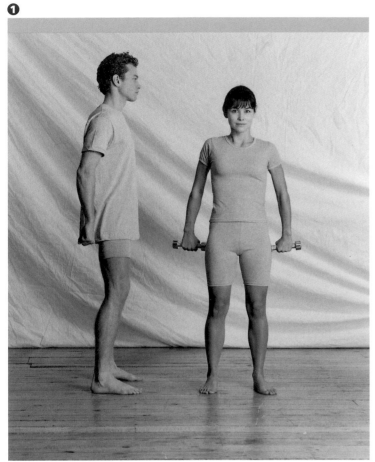

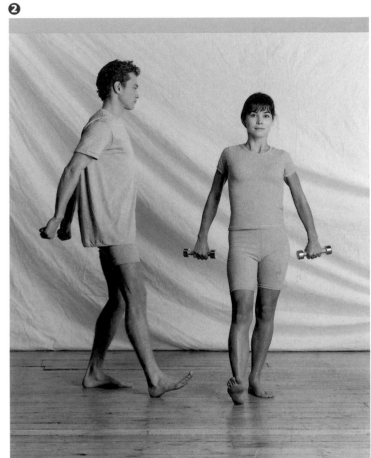

Press back and heel digs

Start with your feet hips' width apart and your arms resting on your buttocks, your hands clenched in loose fists (1). As you step forward with your right leg, touching your heel to the floor in front of you, push both arms straight back behind you (2). As your feet come together again, your arms should come back toward your body.

It might seem more natural to lift your arms in front of your body since your legs are moving forward, but making different demands on your body will keep your mind engaged and help you to improve your coordination.

You can increase the challenge by holding weights, or by bending your standing knee as you step the other leg forward.

Curl-up and reverse curl

By combining these two exercises, you will give your abdominal muscles a comprehensive workout.

For the curl-up, lie on your back with your knees bent and your feet on the floor, and place your hands on your thighs. Tighten your stomach muscles to close the gap between your back and the floor, then contract your stomach muscles to lift your upper back, shoulders, and head (1). With control, lower your upper body to the floor and, just before you get to a position where you feel you can relax, contract your stomach muscles again.

For the reverse curl, keep your hands by your side, your palms turned up. Bring your knees toward your chest, crossing your ankles, and allow your lower back to press into the floor. As you contract your abdominals, your hips will lift up and forward and your knees will move toward your shoulders (2). Release your abdominals in a slow, controlled manner.

For fun, devise different patterns of these two exercises in combination. For example, you could do eight curl-ups and eight reverse curls, then four of each, two of each, one of each. Or try doing them at the same time as an abdominal crunch, repeating this eight times.

As an advanced variation, you can hold your weights close to your ears or on your chest, if you are ready to increase your workload.

❶

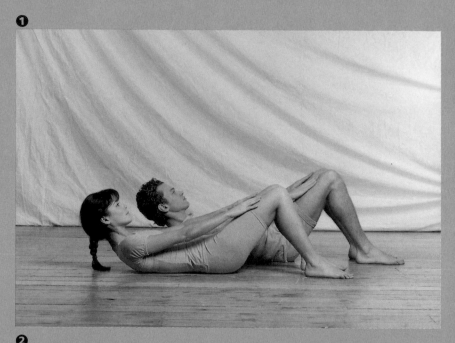

❷

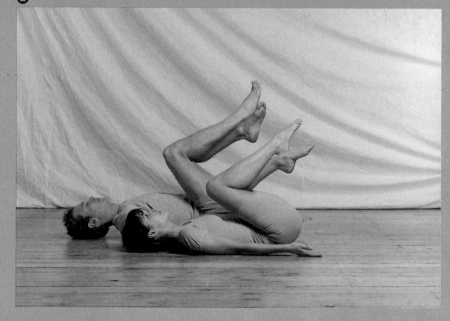

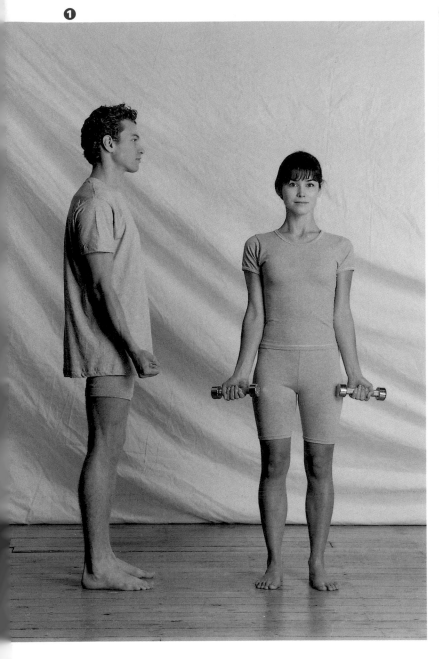

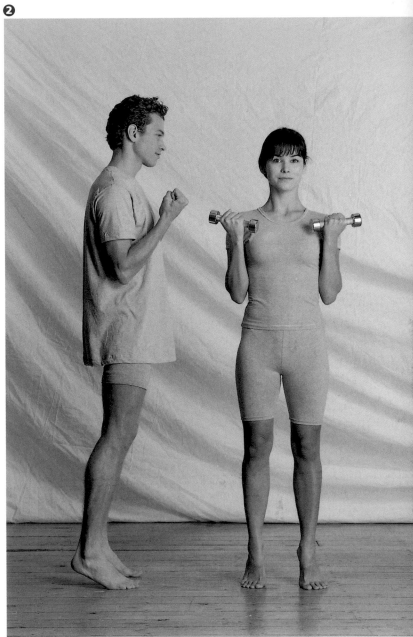

Bicep curl and calf raise

Begin with your feet hips' width apart, and your arms in front of your thighs with hands clenched in loose fists (1). As you raise yourself onto your toes to strengthen your calf muscles, bend your elbows and bring your palms up and in toward your shoulders (2). Lower your arms as you lower your heels. As a variation, you can use weights or lift one leg off the floor.

Index

Acknowledgments

Illustrations: Marks Creative

Additional text: Sara Black

Proofreader: Phyllida Hancock

Indexer: Clare Richards

Chair: Montego, by Habitat

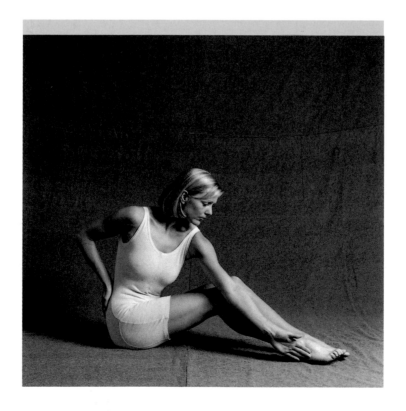